SALIVARY GLAND PATHOLOGIES

SALIVARY GLAND PATHOLOGIES

Editors
Nisheet Anant Agni MDS
Assistant Professor
Department of Oral and Maxillofacial Surgery
Sharad Pawar Dental College
Datta Meghe Institute of Medical Sciences
(Deemed University)
Nagpur, Maharashtra, India

Rajiv Mukund Borle MDS FIAOMS
Professor and Head
Department of Oral and Maxillofacial Surgery
Sharad Pawar Dental College
Datta Meghe Institute of Medical Sciences
(Deemed University)
Nagpur, Maharashtra, India

Foreword
Vedprakash Mishra

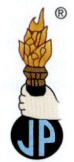

JAYPEE BROTHERS MEDICAL PUBLISHERS (P) LTD
New Delhi • London • Philadelphia • Panama

Jaypee Brothers Medical Publishers (P) Ltd.

Headquarters
Jaypee Brothers Medical Publishers (P) Ltd.
4838/24, Ansari Road, Daryaganj
New Delhi 110 002, India
Phone: +91-11-43574357
Fax: +91-11-43574314
Email: jaypee@jaypeebrothers.com

Overseas Offices
J.P. Medical Ltd.
83, Victoria Street, London
SW1H 0HW (UK)
Phone: +44-2031708910
Fax: +02-03-0086180
Email: info@jpmedpub.com

Jaypee-Highlights Medical Publishers Inc.
City of Knowledge, Bld. 237, Clayton
Panama City, Panama
Phone: +507-301-0496
Fax: +507-301-0499
Email: cservice@jphmedical.com

Jaypee Brothers Medical Publishers Ltd.
The Bourse
111, South Independence Mall East
Suite 835, Philadelphia, PA 19106, USA
Phone: + 267-519-9789
Email: joe.rusko@jaypeebrothers.com

Jaypee Brothers Medical Publishers (P) Ltd.
17/1-B Babar Road, Block-B, Shaymali
Mohammadpur, Dhaka-1207
Bangladesh
Mobile: +08801912003485
Email: jaypeedhaka@gmail.com

Jaypee Brothers Medical Publishers (P) Ltd.
Shorakhute, Kathmandu
Nepal
Phone: +00977-9841528578
Email: jaypee.nepal@gmail.com

Website: www.jaypeebrothers.com
Website: www.jaypeedigital.com

© 2013, Jaypee Brothers Medical Publishers

All rights reserved. No part of this book may be reproduced in any form or by any means without the prior permission of the publisher.

Inquiries for bulk sales may be solicited at: jaypee@jaypeebrothers.com

This book has been published in good faith that the contents provided by the contributors contained herein are original, and is intended for educational purposes only. While every effort is made to ensure accuracy of information, the publisher and the editors specifically disclaim any damage, liability, or loss incurred, directly or indirectly, from the use or application of any of the contents of this work. If not specifically stated, all figures and tables are courtesy of the editors. Where appropriate, the readers should consult with a specialist or contact the manufacturer of the drug or device.

Salivary Gland Pathologies

First Edition: **2013**

ISBN: 978-93-80704-72-2

Printed at: S. Narayan & Sons

Dedicated to
Our parents, Teachers
Colleagues and all our patients

— *Nisheet Anant Agni*
— *Rajiv Mukund Borle*

Contributors

Samarth Shukla MD DNB
Assistant Professor
Department of General Pathology
Jawaharlal Nehru Medical College
Datta Meghe Institute of Medical Sciences
(Deemed University)
Nagpur, Maharashtra, India

Suhas Jajoo MS MCh (Plastic Surgery)
Professor and Head
Department of Plastic Surgery
Jawaharlal Nehru Medical College
Datta Meghe Institute of Medical Sciences
(Deemed University)
Nagpur, Maharashtra, India

Sujit Vasant Mahajan MDS
Consultant
Oral and Maxillofacial Surgeon
Private Practice
Mumbai, Maharashtra, India

Sunita Vagha MD
Professor and Head
Department of General Pathology
Jawaharlal Nehru Medical College
Datta Meghe Institute of Medical Sciences
(Deemed University)
Nagpur, Maharashtra, India

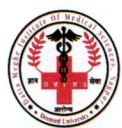

DATTA MEGHE INSTITUTE OF MEDICAL SCIENCES
[Deemed University]
(NAAC Accredited Grade 'A')

Regd. Office: Atrey Layout, Pratap Nagar, NAGPUR-440 022, Maharashtra (India). Ph. 0712-3956552, 3953764, Fax-0712-22455318, E-mail– info@dmims.org, Website-dmims.org
Camp Office: Sawangi (Meghe), Wardha-442 004, Maharashtra (India). Ph. 07152-243542, 240129, 245968, Fax– 07152-244254, Email– medical_wda@sancharnet.in

Dr. Vedprakash Mishra
Vice-Chancellor

डॉ. वेदप्रकाश मिश्रा
कुलगुरू

Foreword

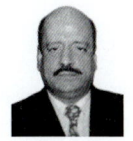

It is heartening to note that Dr Rajiv Mukund Borle, Professor and Head, Department of Oral and Maxillofacial Surgery and Dr Nisheet Anant Agni, Assistant Professor, Department of Oral and Maxillofacial Surgery, Sharad Pawar Dental College, Datta Meghe Institute of Medical Sciences (Deemed University), Nagpur, Maharashtra, India, have authored the book *Salivary Gland Pathologies*.

Their efforts are significantly appreciable, in as much as, it is the end result of their creative and inquisitive, initiative, blended with untiring labor and the single-minded commitment to the cause.

This book indeed is a beautiful compilation of epidemiology, etiology, surgical anatomy, clinical presentation, surgical pathology and their management, pertaining to salivary glands. The book also deals in regard to the various non-neoplastic disorders that afflicts salivary glands along with techniques and modalities of the management.

The another significant and praiseworthy aspect of the book is the extensive number of clinical photographs of different salivary glands pathologies that have been incorporated, which is bound to facilitate the understanding of the issue in a genuine way.

Creative contributions of such a magnitude are not just an end result of a passionate day-dreaming, but are consequence of a deep-rooted commitment and the quest to bring out the best.

The topic chosen for the book is significant, in as much as, the various aspects, with reference to the pathologies of the salivary glands, have been dealt with not only adequately, but also in a very lucid and free-flowing manner. The language availed is easily decipherable and the 'informational inclusions' definitely are bound to satisfy the students and readers alike in more than one way.

It is a book, which can be said to be 'handy, readable, informative' and capable of stating various facets of inquisitive mind and intellect alike.

I unhesitatingly record my sense of appreciation for the authors for their diligent efforts which would be validated exclusively by the appreciation that will evoke from amongst its readers.

Vedprakash Mishra

Preface

It is a proud moment for us to present a comprehensive compilation on salivary gland pathologies. The book is an outcome of a vast compilation of data, both literature-wise and clinical, regarding the various conditions afflicting the salivary glands. Salivary gland disorders are routinely encountered in our day-to-day clinical practice.

The scope of oral and maxillofacial surgery is ever expanding and is no more limited to just minor oral surgical work or extractions. Various pathologic and traumatic conditions affecting the soft and hard tissues of the face now come under the purview of the oral and maxillofacial surgeon.

Salivary gland pathologies include a wide range of disorders ranging from infective to neoplastic. Patients with salivary gland afflictions may present to anyone including a dentist, routine family physician or a surgeon. Prompt diagnosis and management is a key factor in maintaining the health-care standards.

The book deals with a thorough and precise, pointwise discussion and compilation of data pertaining to the relevant surgical anatomy, classification, clinical presentation, management and complications of various salivary gland diseases. It is supported by explicit sketches and illustrations, line diagrams and above all, clinical pictures of most of the conditions affecting salivary glands.

We hope that this small effort of ours helps not only undergraduate and postgraduate students but also to all the clinicians who deal with the diagnosis and management of these disorders.

Nisheet Anant Agni
Rajiv Mukund Borle

Acknowledgments

We wish to express our sincere gratitude to our parents who have been a constant source of inspiration and strength throughout our life and whose constant encouragement, support and blessings have led to the completion of this compilation.

We express our sincere thanks to our mentor Dr Suhas Jajoo, Professor and Head, Department of Plastic Surgery, Jawaharlal Nehru Medical College, Datta Meghe Institute of Medical Sciences (Deemed University), Nagpur, Maharashtra, India, for his guidance, meticulous attention and constant encouragement for the perfection of this work. We are greatly indebted to him for his support throughout this endeavor.

We also thank Dr GSV Prasad, Professor and all other teaching staff, senior and junior colleagues from the Department of Oral and Maxillofacial Surgery, Sharad Pawar Dental College, for their help and support. We especially wish to appreciate the help and assistance of Dr Abhilasha, Senior Lecturer, Department of Oral and Maxillofacial Surgery, for her great help and support throughout.

We also thank Mr Kombe, our artist, who has helped us with the sketches.

We shall be lacking in our duty if we fail to express gratitude to Dr Anita Borges, Consultant Surgical Pathologist and former faculty at the Tata Memorial Hospital, Mumbai, Maharashtra, India, who has not only motivated us but also inspired us to write the book.

Above all we are thankful to all the patients visiting our department without whose inclusion, this final product in the current form would not have been possible.

We also thank all those who have helped us in this endeavor but their names have been unintentionally omitted.

Contents

1. **Introduction** — 1
2. **Embryological Development** — 4
3. **Applied Surgical Anatomy** — 6
   - Parotid gland 6
   - Submandibular glands 21
   - Sublingual glands 25
4. **Historical Perspective** — 29
5. **Classifications** — 31
   - General Classification of Salivary Gland Diseases 31
6. **Diagnosis and Diagnostic Aids** — 34
   - History 34
   - Physical examination 35
   - Parotid tumors 35
   - Submandibular gland tumors 37
   - Sublingual salivary gland 38
   - Minor salivary glands 38
   - Diagnostic aids 40
7. **Non-neoplastic Diseases** — 54
   - Acute bacterial sialadenitis 54
   - Chronic bacterial sialadenitis 62
   - Obstructive disorders of the salivary glands 63
   - Sialolithiasis 64
   - Viral infections of salivary glands 70
   - Non-infectious inflammatory diseases 74
   - Cystic conditions 80
   - Mucoceles 80
   - Ranula 82
   - Salivary fistula 84
8. **Etiology and Pathogenesis of Tumors** — 90
   - Pathophysiology of salivary gland tumors 92
9. **Incidence of Salivary Gland Neoplasms** — 95
10. **Histogenesis of Salivary Gland Neoplasms** — 97
    - Histogenetic concepts 97

11. Surgical Pathology of Salivary Gland Neoplasms — 102
- Surgical pathology   105
- Pleomorphic adenoma   105
- Warthin's Tumor   113
- Oncocytoma   117
- Monomorphic adenoma   120
- Ductal papilloma   125
- Malignant tumors of salivary glands   131
- Adenoid cystic carcinoma   142
- Acinic cell adenocarcinoma   147
- Malignant mixed tumor   152
- Primary squamous cell carcinoma   158
- Clear cell carcinoma   160
- Epithelial–myoepithelial carcinoma   162
- Undifferentiated carcinomas   164

12. Surgical Management of Parotid Neoplasms — 175
- Patient preparation   175
- Skin incision and exposure of the gland   176
- Identification of the facial nerve   180
- Tumor resection   180
- Reconstruction   195

13. Surgical Management of Submandibular and Sublingual Neoplasms — 198
- Incision for access to submandibular gland   198
- Incision for excision of sublingual gland   198
- Extra capsular excision of the submandibular salivary gland   199

14. Surgical Management of Minor Salivary Gland Neoplasms — 203
- Partial maxillectomy   206
- Total maxillectomy   207

15. Complications of Salivary Gland Surgery — 212
- Hematoma   212
- Trismus   212
- Salivary fistula   213
- Facial nerve paresis or paralysis   213
- Auriculotemporal syndrome of frey   214
- Sensory abnormalities associated with greater auricular nerve sacrifice   215

16. Chemotherapy and Radiotherapy — 216
- Chemotherapy in management of salivary gland neoplasms   218

Index   *221*

Introduction

chapter 1

Salivary glands may be classified as major and minor glands. Major glands are paired glands. They include parotid, submandibular and sublingual salivary glands. There are numerous minor salivary glands that are widely distributed of oral cavity of submucous layer. They include labial, buccal, palatine, lingual and incisive glands. All these glands secrete saliva, which serves as a lubricant for the food bolus and has immunologic, digestive and cleansing properties. Based on their secretions, salivary glands are classified as:
1. Mucous salivary glands
2. Serous salivary glands
3. Mixed salivary glands.

Salivary glands are often involved in a wide variety of disorders that frequently require surgical treatment. These glands can be involved with acute and chronic inflammatory processes, give rise to benign and malignant neoplasms, manifest congenital abnormalities or represent involvement of a systemic disorder. Amongst all the disorders, the most common are problems with neoplasms and infections.

Salivary gland disorders can be broadly classified as follows:
1. Developmental anomalies
2. Enlargement of gland
    - Inflammatory
    - Non-inflammatory
3. Cysts
4. Tumors of salivary glands
5. Necrotizing sialometaplasia
6. Salivary gland dysfunction

Salivary glands are susceptible to numerous systemic and local inflammatory conditions, usually secondary to bacterial or viral infections or obstructive pathologies. Trauma to the gland or duct may also result into inflammation. Inflammation of the duct progresses through stages of edema, cellulitis and eventually obstruction. The obstructive phase causes degeneration of glandular parenchyma and fibrosis and hence may often require surgical management.[1]

Tumors of the salivary glands can affect both, the major and minor salivary glands. Salivary gland tumors are uncommon and 95.4% are parenchymal in origin where as 4.6% are interstitial in origin. Interstitial tumors arise from the vessels, lymph nodes and nerves. They could be either benign or malignant. Benign parenchymal salivary gland tumors include pleomorphic adenoma, Warthin's tumor, basal cell adenoma, canalicular adenoma, oxyphilic adenoma, ductal papilloma and myoepithelioma. Malignant salivary gland tumors include mucoepidermoid carcinoma, adenoid cystic carcinoma, acinic cell carcinoma and malignant mixed tumor. Malignant tumors can affect both minor as well as major salivary glands. In most parts of the world the incidence of benign and malignant neoplasms of the salivary glands varies from 1 to 2 per 100,000 populations per year. The majority of lesions occur in the parotid gland. The parotid gland is most commonly involved in neoplasia followed by submandibular gland, minor salivary glands and lastly the sublingual gland. The frequency of occurrence of malignant salivary gland neoplasms is parotid, 25%; submandibular gland, 25%; sublingual gland, 100%; accessory glands, 50% or more.[2] Thus, parotid is the most commonly affected gland by the tumors and a tumor in the minor salivary gland is most likely to be malignant. However, in a survey carried out by Potdar GG and Paymaster JC at Tata Memorial Hospital, Mumbai during 1941 to 1965, it was found that out of 355 salivary gland tumors 110 (31%) were located in minor salivary glands.[2]

Until 1953, there was much confusion regarding histologic and biologic behavior of salivary gland neoplasms, which led to poor management of these neoplasms. Despite their characteristically pronounced variation in histological appearance, all salivary gland tumors were simplistically separated only into 'infiltrating' and 'encapsulated' types. Serious attempts at a clinicopathological correlation were not made until the late 1940s and early 1950s. Foote and Frazell's monograph on tumors of major salivary glands in 1953 was the first ever classification of salivary gland tumors wherein emphasis was placed on histologic classification and analysis of several tumor types under conditions in which surgical treatment was accented. They reviewed 877 cases accumulated over a period of 20 years ending in 1949.[3] Refinement of clinical examination, diagnostic imaging techniques, microscopic diagnosis and immunohistochemical techniques has resulted in more precise diagnosis and treatment.

Salivary gland neoplasms, both benign and malignant, present as painless masses and hence diagnosis of these tumors is essential at an early stage to rule out possibility of a malignancy that could have a poor prognosis.

The management of salivary gland tumors chiefly includes surgical excision of the lesion with or without removal of adjoining structures depending on the histopathological diagnosis of the tumor. Radiotherapy has also been used as an adjunct in the management of high-grade malignant tumors of the salivary glands. The more aggressive surgical approach in the fifth decade of the last century could be attributed to the more precise surgery in regard to the facial nerve exposure and to a centralization of salivary gland tumor treatment in medical centers.

References

1. Rankow RM, Polayes IM. Inflammatory disorders. Surgical Management. Diseases of Salivary glands. WB Saunders, Philadelphia. 1976;9(2):229-38.
2. I Van Der Waal. Salivary gland neoplasms. I Van Der Waal, Prabhu SR, Wilson DF, Daftary DK, Johnson NW (Eds). Oral diseases in the Tropics, Oxford University Press, Delhi. 1993;41:478-86.
3. Carlson ER. Salivary Gland tumors: classification, histogenesis and general considerations. Oral and Maxillofacial surgery clinics of North America. 1995;7(3):519-27.

Embryological development

chapter 2

According to studies that have been conducted on lower mammalian forms such as the rat, the major salivary gland development begins at the end of 2nd week of intrauterine life. The formation of the parotid gland lags behind the sublingual and submandibular glands throughout the prenatal period and is the least developed at birth.[1]

The salivary glands arise from the epithelial lining of the mouth.[2] They arise as a proliferation of oral epithelial cells forming a focal thickening that grows into the underlying ectomesenchyme. Continued growth results in the formation of a small bud connected to the surface by a trailing cord of epithelial cells, with mesenchymal cells condensing around the bud. Clefts develop in the bud, forming two or more new buds and this process is continued and is known as branching morphogenesis. This produces successive generations of buds and a hierarchical ramification of the gland.

Several factors control the branch points and the overall structure of the glands. Members of the fibroblast growth factor protein family along with transforming growth factor b play a major role in the branching. The differential contraction of actin filaments at the basal and apical ends of the epithelial cells probably provides the physical mechanism underlying cleft formation. The deposition of extra-cellular matrix components within the clefts apparently serves to stabilize them. The specific mesenchyme associated with the salivary glands seems to provide the optimum environment for gland development.

The development of lumen within the branched epithelium occurs first in the distal end of the main cord and in branch cords, then in proximal end of the main cord and finally in the central portion of the main cord. Lumina form within the ducts before they develop within the terminal buds. A few studies have hypothesized that apoptosis of centrally located cells in the cell cords may be responsible for lumen formation.

Following the development of the lumen in the terminal buds, the epithelium consists of two layers of cells. The cells of the inner layer differentiate into secretory cells of the mature gland. They may be mucous or serous depending on the gland type. Few cells of the outer layer form contractile myoepithelial cells that are present around the secretory end pieces and intercalated ducts. As the epithelial parenchymal component increases in size and number, there is a decrease in the associated mesenchyme. However, a thin layer of connective tissue remains around each secretory end piece and duct of the adult gland. Thicker partitions of connective tissue (septa) which are continuous with the capsule invest the excretory ducts and divide the gland into lobes and lobules. They contain the nerves and blood vessels which supply the gland.

The parotid gland is the first to appear and begins development at 4th to 6th week of intrauterine life. They develop from the buds that arise from the oral ectodermal lining near the angle of the stomodeum and later grow towards the ear. Ducts form by 10 weeks. Secretion commences by 18 weeks. The capsule and connective tissue develop from the surrounding mesenchyme.

The submandibular glands appear late in the sixth week. They develop from the endodermal buds in the floor of the stomodeum. Acini begin forming at 12 weeks and secretory activity begins at 16 weeks. Growth continues after birth. The sublingual glands appear in the eight week. They develop from endodermal buds in the paralingual sulcus. The minor salivary glands too develop at eight to twelve weeks of gestation.

The cells of the secretory end pieces and ducts attain maturity during last two weeks of intrauterine life. The glands continue to grow postnatally with the volume proportion of acinar tissue increasing and that of ducts, connective tissue and vascular tissue decreasing up to two years of life.

References

1. Batsakis JG. Tumors of the head and neck – Clinical and pathological considerations. Williams and Wilkins, Baltimore. 1979;2(1)
2. Hand AR. Salivary Glands. Nanci A (Ed). Ten Cate's Oral Histology-Development, Structure and function. Mosby, Missouri. 2005;11:299-328.

Applied surgical anatomy

chapter 3

A salivary gland is any cell or organ discharging a secretion into the oral cavity.[1] Salivary glands are classified into major and minor salivary glands. Major salivary glands are paired glands and include parotid, submandibular (Submaxillary) and sublingual glands (Bartholin's gland). They are located at some distance from the oral mucosa with which they connect by extraglandular ducts. Minor salivary glands lie in the mucosa or sub mucosa opening directly through mucosa or indirectly via many short ducts and include anterior glands of the tongue, numerous small lingual glands (including von Ebner's glands) and small labial, buccal and palatal glands. Their function is lubrication of food to assist deglutition, moistening of buccal mucosa, aiding speech, providing an aqueous medium necessary for perception of taste, as a fluid seal for sucking and suckling, secretion of digestive enzymes – salivary amylase and hormones and other compounds such as glucagon – like protein (Lawrence et al 1977)[1] and serotonin (Feryter 1961)[1] and secretion of antimicrobial agents – SIgA and lysozyme.

The rate of secretion of individual glands ranges from barely perceptible during sleep to as high as 4 ml/min on maximal stimulation. In a 24 hour period, the submandibular gland produces 70% of the saliva, parotid gland 25% and minor glands another 5%.[2]

Parotid gland

They are the largest of the salivary glands weighing approximately about 15–30 grams (Average 25 grams).[1] It is an irregular, lobulated, yellowish mass lying largely below the external acoustic meatus in a deep hollow between the mandible and sternocleidomastoid muscle.

Extent of the gland (Figure 3.1)

Bulk of the gland lies in the retromandibular fossa and reaches medially to the styloid process and muscles arising from it. Superiorly it extends up to external acoustic meatus, which is situated in a groove of the gland. Superiorly, the gland reaches posteriorly to the mastoid process and sternocleidomastoid muscle. Anteriorly, it is in contact with the posterior border of medial pterygoid muscle and mandibular ramus. A part of the gland extends anteriorly on the outer surface of the mandibular ramus and Masseter muscle as thin, triangular layer[3] which may cover the TMJ in front

Applied surgical anatomy 7

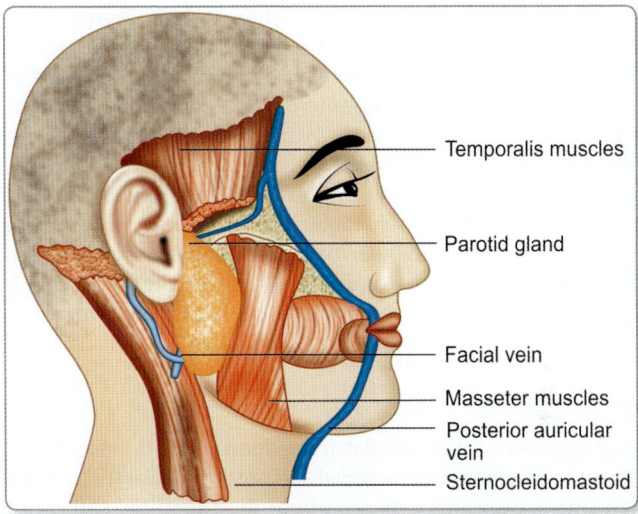

Figure 3.1 Extent of parotid gland

of the ear but never extends beyond the lower border of the zygomatic arch.

Capsule

The parotid gland is surrounded by a connective tissue capsule. In addition, it has a dense fibrous capsule derived from the investing layer of the deep cervical fascia, which posteriorly surrounds the sternocleidomastoid muscle and anteriorly overlies the masseter and incompletely invests the gland. The capsule is tight and firmly connected with strong septa dividing the lobes and lobules of the gland from one another. The surface component of the parotid fascia is attached to the zygomatic arch and is exceedingly tough and unyielding. The result is building of immense pressure within the capsule and hence parotid space infections are extremely tender but show minimal swelling. Early incision and drainage is the treatment of choice in parotid infections even if there is no fluctuation in order to relieve the pressure to avoid further parenchymal damage. So also, there is an inherent anatomical weakness in the capsule covering the deep surface of the gland adjacent to the loose areolar tissues of the lateral pharyngeal wall resulting into spread of a parotid abscess into the lateral pharyngeal space, if not drained promptly.[3a]

In addition, benign tumors are slow to project outwards to any great extent and hence take years to present as unsightly bulges. The facial nerve is often displaced inwards by the tumor, where there is less resistance from the deep component of the parotid fascia or upwards and downwards, depending on its relation to the tumor.

As it extends medially over the anteromedial and posteromedial aspects of the gland it thins out progressively. Medial to the gland it is attached to the styloid process, mandible and tympanic plate blending with fibrous sheaths of related muscles. Fascial thickening extends from styloid process to the mandibular angle and forms stylomandibular ligament, which separates parotid gland from submandibular gland, denoting their development from 1st and 2nd branchial arches, respectively. It is fused at the anterior border of sternocleidomastoid muscle and its fascia but isolated from the other structures by thin layers of connective tissue.

Gland morphology (Figure 3.2)

Parotid gland is like an inverted, flat, three sided pyramid, presenting a small superior and superficial, anteromedial and posteromedial surfaces. It tapers inferiorly into a blunt apex. As seen from the superficial surface, parotid gland is roughly wedge shaped. If cut across in a horizontal plane, it would also be found to be wedge shaped with its base in the lateral position and its apex against the pharyngeal wall.

The gland chiefly consists of a larger superficial and smaller deep lobes divided by the facial nerve and its branches which pass forward within the parotid gland for a variable but short distance. 80% of the parotid gland lies superficial to the nerve, thus comprising the bulk of the gland and 20% of the gland lies deep to the nerve entering the parapharyngeal space. A narrow isthmus connects the superficial and deep lobes. The superficial and deep lobes are separated by the posterior surface of the ramus of the

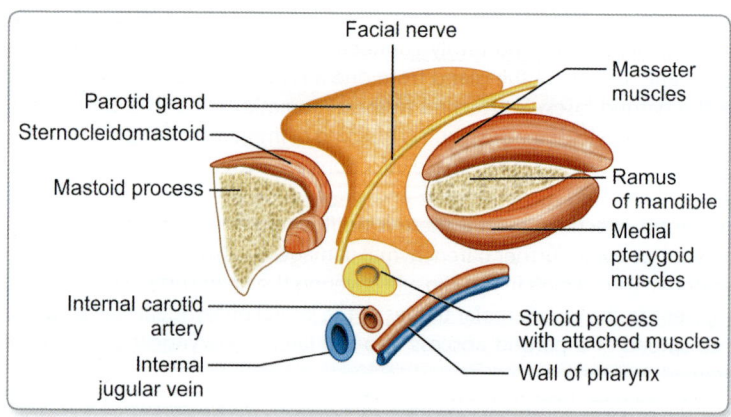

Figure 3.2 Transverse section of parotid gland

mandible. Most commonly neoplasm develops in the superficial lobe of the parotid gland. However, when both the lobes of the gland are involved by tumor, the classical appearance is described as dumbbell shaped tumor **(Figure 3.3)**.

Isthmus is most often found in the bifurcation of the facial nerve into upper temporofacial and lower cervicofacial divisions **(Figure 3.4)**.

McWhorter described these two divisions of the facial nerve as passing between superficial and deep parts on either side of an isthmus. According to his description the superficial and deep parts of the gland thus form lobes that are usually distinct and readily separable and have separate duct

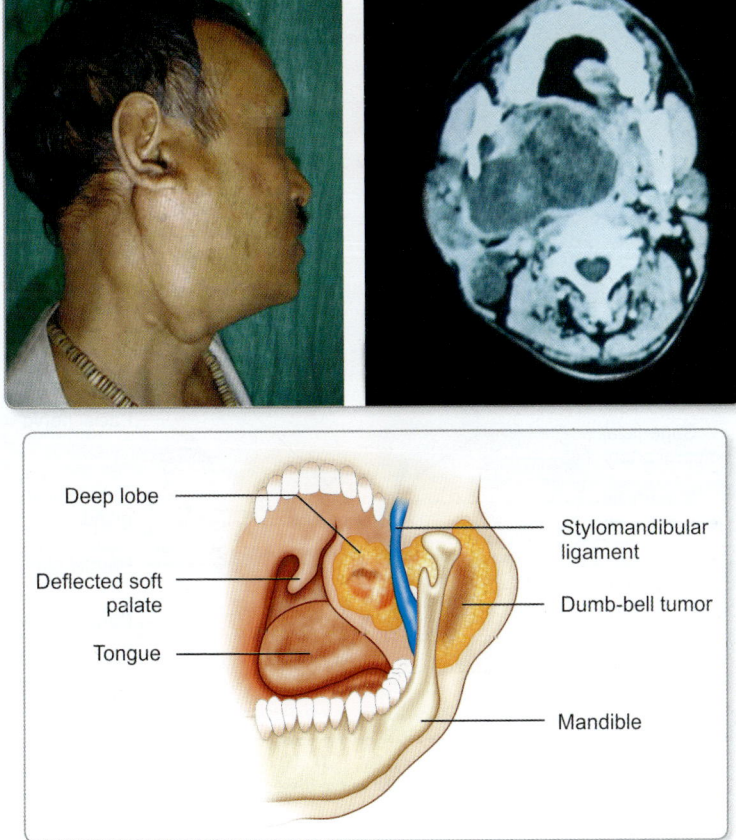

Figure 3.3 Dumb-bell tumor of parotid gland

10 Salivary gland pathologies

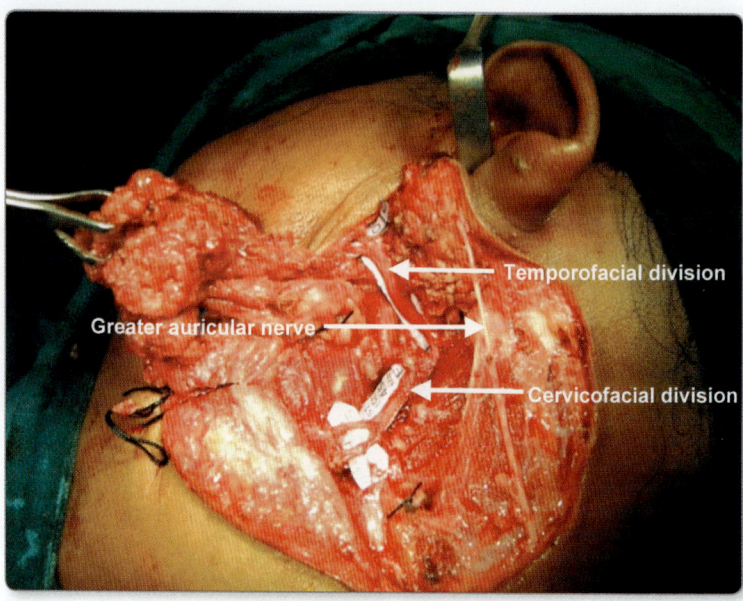

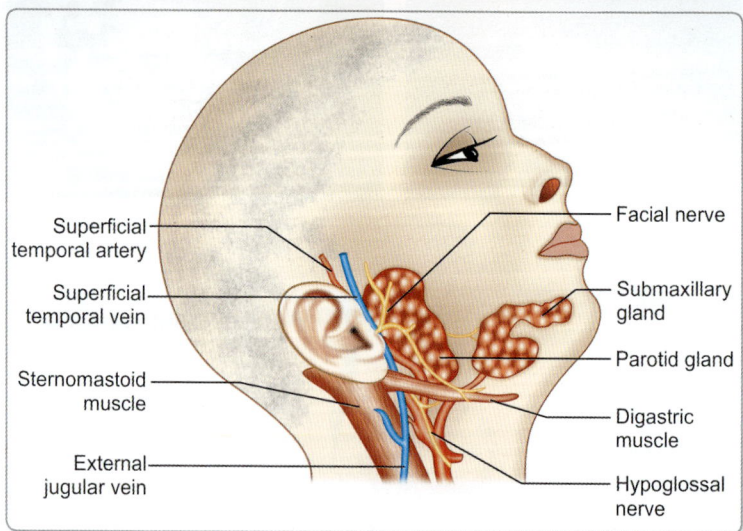

Figure 3.4 Facial nerve dissection

systems, except where they are united by an isthmus. Thus according to this description the facial nerve does not traverse the gland but the lobes are folded about the nerve.[4]

The facial nerve is related to the parotid gland in a number of ways.[4] **(Figure 3.5)**.

a. Superficial and deep lobes united above, so that gland is essentially folded over the nerve.
b. The two lobes united by an isthmus.
c. Combination of (a) and (b)
d. According to McKenzie, gland and nerve intertwined within superficial and deep lobes, relation varying according to plane of section.

The intratemporal and intraparotid facial nerve has varied pattern of branching which is of immense surgical importance. Detailed studies of the intratemporal course of the facial nerve have demonstrated both bifurcation and trifurcation of the main trunk within the mastoid segment. This intratemporal division of the facial nerve is associated with congenital abnormalities of the pinna or inner ear.[5]

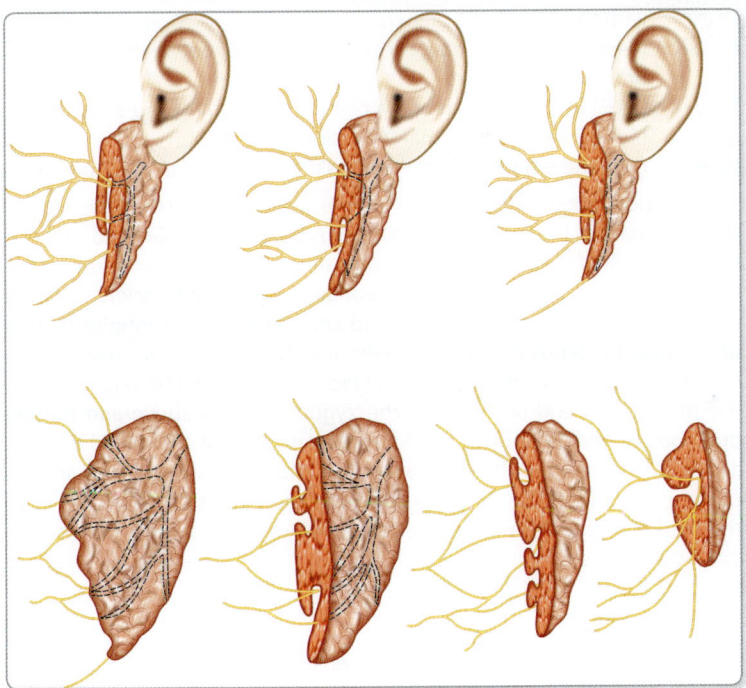

Figure 3.5 Relation of facial nerve with parotid gland
(*Source:* Hollinshead WH. The Face. Anatomy for Surgeons: Vol I. The Head and Neck)

Katz and Catalano, 1987, demonstrated evidence of double trunked facial nerve trunks in three out of hundred cases of parotidectomies.[6] Detailed study of the intra-temporal course of facial nerve has demonstrated both bifurcation and trifurcation of the facial nerve trunk within the mastoid segment. Division of the facial nerve within the temporal bone is frequently associated with congenital abnormalities of the pinna or inner ear.

Davis et al, 1956 had classified the branching pattern of the facial nerve into six types followed by Miehlke, Stennert and Chilla, 1979 who classified the branching pattern of the facial nerve into eight types. More recently, Katz and Catalano, 1987 reclassified the branching patterns of the facial nerve into five types based on operative findings as against the previous studies based on cadaveric dissections.[5] The five types of branching patterns are as follows **(Figure 3.6)**:

Type 1: (25%) This pattern lacks anastomotic links between the main branches of each division. In one subtype there is splitting and subsequent reunion of the Zygomatic branch while in the other the mandibular branch splits and reunites.

Type 2: (14%) In this type subdivisions of the buccal branch fuse distally with the Zygomatic branch.

Type 3: (44%) There are major communications between the buccal branches and others.

Type 4: (14%) In this type there is a complex branching and anastomotic pattern between the major divisions.

Type 5: (3%) The facial nerve leaves the skull as more than one trunk.

Superior margin of the gland extends upwards, behind the TMJ, into the posterior part of the mandibular fossa. This part is called 'Glenoid process'. Inferior corner of the gland extends below the level of the lower border of the mandible in the space between mandibular angle and sternocleidomastoid muscle. This inferior extension is called 'cervical lobe'. The anterior margin of the gland extends forwards superficial to the Masseter muscle to form the 'facial process'.[7] A small part of the facial process may be separate from the main gland and lie between the zygomatic arch above and parotid duct below and is known as the accessory part of the gland or pars accessoria or socia parotidis. The accessory lobe is present in less than 50% of the population.[8] The deep part of the gland extends forward between the medial pterygoid muscle and the ramus of the mandible to form the 'pterygoid process'.[7]

Parotid duct

It is also known as Stensen's duct (**Figure 3.1**). It is about 5 cms (2 inches) long and passes forward across the masseter about a finger breadth below the zygomatic arch.[7] It begins with the confluence of two main tributaries

Applied surgical anatomy 13

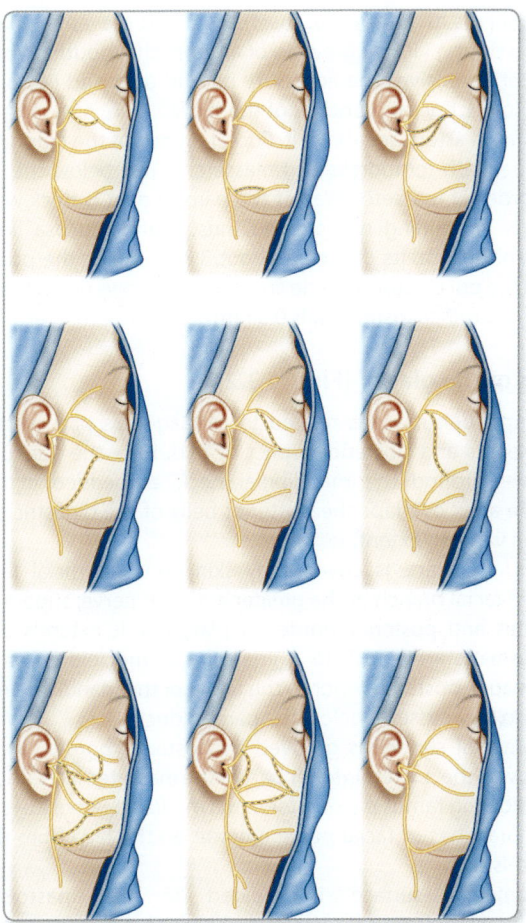

Figure 3.6 Katz – Catlano classification based on operative findings
(*Source:* Adapted from Cawson R, Gleeson M. Anatomy and physiology of the salivary glands. Gleeson M. Editor. Scott-Brown's Otolaryngology. Basic sciences)

within the anterior part of the gland, and then crosses the masseter at junction of upper and middle 1/3rd. At its anterior border it turns medially almost at right angle, traversing the corpus adiposum (Buccal fat pad of Bichat/Suctorial pad of infants)[3] and the buccinator muscle. It then runs obliquely forwards for a short distance between the buccinator and oral mucosa to open upon a small papilla opposite the crown of 2nd maxillary molar. The oblique passage of the duct forwards between the mucosa and buccinator serves as a valve like mechanism and prevents inflation of the duct system during violent blowing of air from the mouth.[7] While crossing the masseter, it receives the accessory parotid duct and lies between the upper and lower buccal branches of the facial nerve. Accessory gland and transverse facial artery are above it. Buccal branch of the mandibular nerve emerging beneath temporalis and masseter is just below the duct at the anterior border of masseter. Wall of the parotid duct is thick with external fibrous layer containing non-striated muscle and mucosa lined by low columnar epithelium. Its caliber is about 3 mm but at the point where it penetrates the buccinators muscle an isthmus narrows down the duct to 1.2 mm and at the orifice (ostium) it is 0.5 mm.[7a]

Relations of the gland[7] (Figure 3.2)

Concave superior surface is related to cartilaginous part of the external acoustic meatus and posterior aspect of TMJ. Here the auriculotemporal nerve curves around the mandibular neck, embedded in the gland's capsule. The apex overlaps the posterior belly of the digastric and carotid triangle to a variable extent.

Superficial surface is covered by skin and superficial fascia which contains the facial branch of the greater auricular nerve, superficial parotid lymph nodes and posterior border of platysma. It extends upwards up to the zygomatic arch, back to overlap the sternocleidomastoid muscle, down to its apex posteroinferior to the angle of the mandible and forwards superficial to the masseter below the parotid duct.

Anteromedial surface is grooved by posterior border of mandibular ramus. It covers the posteroinferior part of the masseter, lateral aspect of the TMJ and adjoining ramus passing forwards medial to ramus to reach medial pterygoid. Branches of facial nerve emerge on the face from the anterior margin of this surface.

Posteromedial surface is molded to the mastoid process, sternocleidomastoid muscle, posterior belly of digastric muscle, styloid process and its muscles. External carotid artery grooves this surface before entering the gland. The internal carotid artery and internal jugular vein are separated from the gland by the styloid process and its muscles. Anteromedial and posteromedial surfaces meet at a medial margin which may project so deeply as to be in contact with the lateral wall of the pharynx.

Structures traversing the gland (Figure 3.2)

Structures traversing the parotid gland from medial to lateral (deep to superficial) are external carotid artery, retromandibular vein and facial nerve. Few members of the parotid group of lymph nodes are also located within the gland.[7]

External carotid artery is covered by the cervical lobe in the retromandibular fossa. It is situated at first in a groove on the medial surface of the gland and eventually enters the posteromedial surface dividing into maxillary artery which emerges from the anteromedial surface and the superficial temporal artery which gives off transverse facial artery in the gland and ascends to leave its upper limit. These branches with their venous counterparts must be ligated when the deep lobe of the gland is removed.

The postauricular artery may also branch from the external carotid artery within the gland leaving by its posteromedial surface.

Retromandibular vein is formed by union of maxillary vein and superficial temporal vein. It traverses superficial to external carotid artery from region of mandibular neck to inferior corner of cervical lobe, i.e. entire gland. It divides into anterior and posterior divisions which join facial vein and posterior auricular vein to form common facial vein and external jugular vein respectively. The retromandibular vein lies in the deep lobe of the gland immediately medial to the facial nerve and its branches, although very occasionally it may be superficial to it. It gives off small tributaries which pass outwards between the nerve branches and which may be a source of troublesome bleeding when dissecting out the nerve.

Most superficial structure is facial nerve which emerges from the fallopian canal and exits from the stylomastoid foramen to pass anteriorly, inferiorly and laterally and enters high on the posteromedial surface of the gland immediately behind the mandibular ramus. It immediately divides into two main divisions, temporofacial and cervicofacial, from which its terminal branches diverge to leave the anteromedial surface passing medial to its anterior margin. The terminal branches of the facial nerve form a plexus which is known as *pes anserinus*.[9] Facial nerve branches in the substance of the gland after crossing the external carotid artery and retromandibular vein on their lateral side. Branches of the facial nerve emerge at the superior, anterior and inferior borders of the gland.

The facial nerve and its branches pass forward within the parotid gland for a variable but short distance and divide it into superficial and deep parts or lobes. 80% of the parotid gland lies superficial to the nerve and 20% of the gland lies deep to the nerve entering the parapharyngeal space. Superficial lobe comprises the bulk of the gland. The superficial and deep lobes are connected by a narrow isthmus. Isthmus is most often found in the bifurcation of the facial nerve.

McWhorter described these two divisions of the facial nerve as passing between superficial and deep parts on either side of an isthmus. According to his description the superficial and deep parts of the gland thus form lobes that are usually distinct and readily separable and have separate duct systems, except where they are united by an isthmus. Thus according to this description the facial nerve does not traverse the gland but the lobes are folded about the nerve.[6]

The facial nerve bisects the gland unequally into a major portion lateral to it and a smaller part medial to it; hence most of the tumors are found superficial to the nerve.[10]

J Mckenzie has stated that this concept of superficial and deep lobes connected by an isthumus and otherwise separated by a plane in which lie the branches of the facial nerve is a simplification that does not actually exist. He found that there were many isthmi between the branches of facial nerve in addition to the isthmus between the two main branches. Each isthmus had ducts joining the deep and superficial part. He gave seven different relations of the facial nerve and the parotid gland.[6]

Blood supply, lymphatics and nerve supply[7]

The external carotid artery and its terminal branches supply the parotid gland. The retromandibular vein drains the gland.

The lymph vessels drain into the parotid lymph nodes and the deep cervical lymph nodes.

Parasympathetic secretomotor fibers from the inferior salivary nucleus of the ninth cranial nerve supply the gland. Nerve fibers pass to the Otic ganglion via the tympanic branch of the Glossopharyngeal nerve and the lesser petrosal nerve. Post-ganglionic parasympathetic fibers reach the parotid gland via the auriculotemporal nerve, which lies in contact with the deep surface of the gland. Postganglionic sympathetic fibers reach the gland as a plexus of nerves around the external carotid artery.

Identification of the facial nerve

The facial nerve can be identified either proximally or distally. Proximally the main trunk of the nerve is identified before it enters the gland. Distally it is identified as branches after the nerve leaves the gland.[11] The facial nerve is spared as far as possible. If this is not possible, the facial nerve should be immediately reconstructed with an interpositional nerve graft.[12] As quoted by Marshall Strome, functioning facial nerves are retained in the presence of any grade malignancy, including nerve encasement by tumor. It is resected only when function is impaired preoperatively.[13] However, Woods JE et al state that the nerve should be sacrificed if there is intra-operative evidence of gross invasion or microscopic infiltration of the nerve by tumor, even in the presence of normal preoperative facial nerve function.[14]

Identification for the preservation of the facial nerve is carried out in three ways:
1. Early direct identification of the main trunk where it exits through the stylomastoid foramen.
2. Retrograde approach to the trunk from either the mandibular branch where it passes over the retromandibular (posterior facial) vein or the peripheral branches alongside the parotid duct.

3. Supravital staining of the parotid gland, contrasting the blue normal gland from the unstained tumor and the gleaming white facial nerve branches.

There are four facial nerve pointers at the stylomastoid foramen.[11] They are as follows:

1. The cartilaginous pointer described by Conley (1978) is an artificially created landmark at its anterior inferior border formed by posterior traction on the external auditory canal. The backward pull on the cartilage causes the meatus to assume the shape of a horn, the curved extremity of which allegedly points to the position of the facial nerve.[11] The nerve is located medial and inferior to the pointer. This is probably the least reliable as it depends on the configuration of the cartilaginous meatus.[15]
2. The segment of the nerve which lies in the interval between the stylomastoid foramen and parotid gland is extremely short, but is an ideal location to find the facial nerve before the parotidectomy commences. It is best found by searching in the tympanomastoid sulcus which is formed by the edge of the bony external meatus on one hand and the anterior face of the mastoid process on the other.[11] The tympanomastoid sulcus lies at the apex of the vaginomastoid angle, which is formed by meeting of the vaginal process of tympanic portion of the temporal bone and mastoid process.[15] The nerve emerges from the stylomastoid foramen some 3–4 mm deep to the outer edge of the bony external canal.[16] However; the groove is filled with fibrofatty lobules that mimic the trunk of the facial nerve which may lie as deep as 1 cm to this landmark.[11]
3. The most reliable landmark for finding the nerve is the posterior belly of the digastric muscle which lies just inferior to the nerve. The anterior superior aspect of the posterior belly of the digastric muscle is inserted just behind the stylomastoid foramen.[11]
4. The styloid process is a useful confirmatory landmark. The facial nerve courses lateral to the styloid process near the base of the styloid. However, to depend on it for finding the nerve is to court trouble since it lies medial and anterior to the point of emergence of the nerve from the mastoid. The posterior auricular artery bleeds frequently while looking for the facial nerve since it lies below and just lateral to the nerve.[11]
5. Length of facial nerve trunk from its bifurcation into upper and lower divisions ranges from 8.6 mm to 22.8 mm with a mean of 14 mm. The most consistent landmark to locate the facial nerve trunk according to study by Pather et al, 2006 is posterior belly of digastric and tragal pointer and transverse process of axis.[17]

18 Salivary gland pathologies

An alternative approach is to remove the mastoid tip. On removal of bone along the medial aspect of mastoid tip along the digastric ridge, the stylomastoid foramen is seen. Alternatively, a complete mastoidectomy can be performed to identify the facial nerve in its vertical course through the mastoid.[15]

Distance of the facial nerve pointers from the surrounding landmarks [17] (Figure 3.7)

S. No.	Pointer	Distance in mm	Mean in mm
1	Tragal pointer	24.3 – 49.2	34
2	Posterior belly of digastric	9.7 – 24.3	14.6
3	External auditory canal	7.3 – 21.9	13.4
4	Tympanomastoid suture	4.9 – 18.6	10.0
5	Styloid process	4.3 – 18.6	9.7
6	Transverse process of axis	9.7 – 36.8	16.9
7	Angle of mandible	25.3 – 48.69	38.1

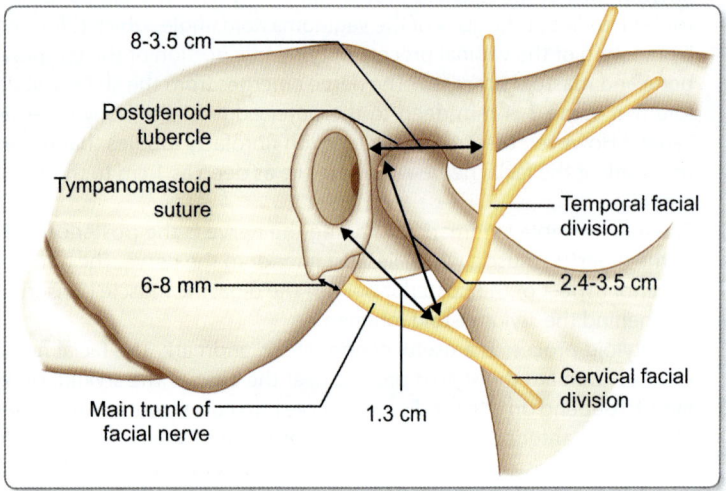

Figure 3.7 Distance from facial nerve pointers
(*Source:* Peter Quinn. Atlas of TMJ surgeries)

In cases where locating the facial nerve trunk is difficult by using the preauricular approach due to distortion of anatomy due to the tumor, the surgeon can locate a peripheral branch of the nerve and trace it proximally. There are very few reports in the literature on retrograde or centripetal identification techniques for isolation of the nerve from its peripheral branches. The easiest branch to locate is the ramus mandibularis. Baker et al, have reported that the ramus mandibularis is located 1 to 2 cm below the inferior border of mandible, based on 2000 parotidectomies. Only in few instances where the tissues were lax, it was located 3 to 4 cm below the inferior border.[15]

Work and Bailey presented several examples of retrograde approach from buccal, mandibular and temporal rami in the parotid gland. Pia F et al[11] recommend following the deep parotid vein as reference for mandibular rami which cross it laterally. Also, they recommend isolation of the orbito-zygomatic nerve as being easier and safer as localization of this branch can always be traced to the anterosuperior emergence of the parotid with an oblique course towards the lateral canthus of the eye. This nerve branch of adequate caliber in its peripheral portion crosses the zygomatic process at an acute angle and since most parotid pathologies develop in the medio-inferior portion of the gland, is easier to identify.[18]

Intraoperative facial nerve monitoring using electromyographic techniques has also been routinely employed for cerebellopontine angle surgery and can also be used for identification of main branch or the peripheral branches in centripetal or retrograde approach.[18] Witt[19] has demonstrated a high rate of facial nerve paralysis in a group monitored during superficial parotidectomy with conclusions that facial nerve monitoring using electromyographic techniques is optional. However, it can play an important and advantageous part in the surgical treatment in recurrent parotid neoplasms.

The proximity of the marginal mandibular branch of the facial nerve to the retromandibular vein at its point of emergence from the tail of the parotid gland provides an alternative method of locating the nerve. The gland that is superficial to the vein is split, looking for the nerve as it crosses superficial to the vein. By working backwards along the nerve the two divisions, the other branches and the main trunk can be found.[15]

The facial nerve can also be located by finding the buccal branch which runs parallel to the zygomatic arch but 1 cm below it. It runs adjacent to the parotid duct, more commonly along the inferior aspect of the duct. According to Peterson et al, the buccal branch is located in the buccal space 5.5 to 6.0 cm in front of the ear lobe.[15]

Farrior et al noted that, in children the facial nerve trunk exits the stylomastoid foramen through the triangle formed by the cartilaginous ear canal, sternocleidomastoid muscle and posterior belly of digastric muscle. The facial nerve trunk can be located approximately 1 cm anterior to the mastoid process and 1.5 cm posterior to the ramus of mandible. The parotid does not extend posterior to the ramus of the mandible in the newborn infant and consequently covers only the lower distal branches of the nerve.[20]

The upper division of the facial nerve, which divides into temporal, upper zygomatic, lower zygomatic and buccal branches, is much stouter than the lower division and therefore can withstand more handling.

In elderly or obese individuals the branches of the facial nerve are often tortuous both mediolaterally and anteroposteriorly, a feature which makes them liable to damage if efforts to keep the tissues constantly on the stretch are neglected while the nerve is being dissected. The lower zygomatic branch invariably lies above the parotid duct, a point to be remembered when attempting to deal with duct stenoses or stones.

The lower division passes downwards and forwards but lacks the outward inclination of the upper division and by comparison therefore lies deeper. The thinness of the branches of the lower division, particularly the mandibular branch, makes paralysis of the depressor anguli oris a common complication of parotidectomy. The very fine interlacing nerve fibers between one branch and another is the reason why the facial nerve withstands more than a modest degree of handling at operation and yet still recover. Communicating branches between lower buccal and mandibular branches are often absent and hence there are increased chances of paralysis of muscles supplied by the marginal mandibular nerve.

Facial nerve monitoring

The goals of facial nerve monitoring are early identification of the nerve, warning the surgeon of any unexpected stimulation, mapping the course of the nerve by using electrical stimulation, reducing trauma to the facial nerve during rerouting or dissection and evaluation and prognosis of facial nerve function at the conclusion of surgery.

There are two types of facial nerve monitoring. The first is EMG. Ipsilateral facial muscle electromyographic activity is used and is continuously displayed into the operating room via a loud speaker. Needle electrodes are placed into the muscle. Electrical activity is sent between a needle electrode pair and this potential difference is displayed on an oscilloscope. Positive feedback occurs in relation to surgical events. There is background baseline white noise and increased EMG activity with either nerve irritation or direct nerve stimulation. This can be used for nerve identification or as a predictor of prognosis.

The other type of monitoring device is pressure or strain gauge sensor. This is a mechanical pressure sensor. It is positioned in the corner of the patient's mouth. It applies light pressure to the facial muscles of the cheek. Muscle contractions cause a change in pressure applied to the sensor. This results in an audible alarm that alerts the surgeon. These are supra-threshold responses that detect actual movement and are less sensitive in the EMG systems.

Facial nerve monitoring can be used in conjunction with the nerve stimulator. Stimulators come in two basic flavors. The first is a monopolar, when current disseminates in all the directions from the tip. This is dependent on the distance of the probe to the nerve as well as the conductive properties of the intervening tissue. The strength of the stimulus necessary is related to the integrity of the nerve. This is very useful in nerve identification. A bipolar stimulator has two probes – the current flow is limited to the region between those two probes. A bipolar stimulator is more precise and it requires closer proximity in alignment to the nerves. While a mono-stimulator is more useful in nerve identification, the bipolar stimulator is more useful if the course of the nerve is evident.

Drawbacks of monitoring
1. It increases the cost.
2. It requires an observer for interpretation and does not prevent direct injury to the nerve from dissection.
3. It is not a very useful adjunct when the nerve and its branches are easily identifiable.

Submandibular glands

It is irregular in shape and of the size of a walnut. It has a mixture of serous and mucous acini, but is chiefly serous. It lies partly under cover of the body of mandible. Although ovoid in appearance when viewed from the lateral direction, it is in fact U-shaped in sagittal section possessing a large superficial and small deep lobe, continuous with each other around the posterior border of the mylohyoid. In operations to remove the gland, the retraction of the mylohyoid forwards will facilitate exposure of the deep part of the gland and duct. The upper pole lies on the medial surface of the mandible in the submandibular fovea and lower pole extends beyond boundaries of the digastric triangle covering intermediate tendon of the digastric muscle. The gland is palpable between the index finger placed on the floor of the mouth and thumb placed anteromedial to the angle of mandible below the floor.

Extent of the gland

Superficial part is situated in the digastric triangle and reaches forward to the anterior belly of the digastric and back to the stylomandibular ligament which separates it from the parotid gland. Superiorly it extends medial to the body of the mandible and inferiorly it approaches the greater cornu of the hyoid which serves as a useful landmark when marking the incision for the operation to remove the gland. Inferiorly it overlaps intermediate tendon of the digastric and the hyoidean attachment of the stylohyoid. It has an inferior, lateral and medial surface.

The deep part of the gland extends forwards to the posterior end of the sublingual gland and lies between the mylohyoid infero-laterally and the hyoglossus and styloglossus medially. Posterior end is continuous with superficial part of the gland around posterior border of the mylohyoid muscle.

Capsule

It is partially enclosed between two layers of deep cervical fascia extending from the hyoid's greater corner – one layer passes to the mandible's lower border covering the gland's inferior surface and the other passes to the mylohyoid line on the medial surface of the mandible and covers medial surface of the gland. In contrast to the parotid capsule, that of the submandibular gland is only loosely attached to the substance of the gland itself because of the loose texture of the interlobar and interlobular connective tissue. Hence the gland can be easily shelled out of the niche.[6]

Relations of the superficial part[12]

The inferolateral surface is covered by skin, platysma, deep fascia and is crossed by facial vein and facial nerve's cervical branch. Near the mandible the submandibular lymph nodes are in contact with the gland and some may be embedded in it. Hence while clearing the submandibular lymph nodes during neck dissection; it is essential to excise the gland along with the nodes as they are adherent to the gland.

The lateral surface is in relation with the submandibular fossa on the medial surface of the mandibular body and the mandibular attachment of the medial pterygoid muscle. Facial artery grooves its posterosuperior part lying at first, deep to the gland and then emerging between its lateral surface and the mandibular attachment of the medial pterygoid to reach the lower border of the mandible. While excising the gland, the facial artery is visualized by retracting the posterior belly of diagastric inferiorly. The artery is seen emerging inferior to the posterior belly of diagastric and ascends superiorly clinging to the inferior part of the submandibular gland. Hence, during excision of the submandibular gland it is essential to ligate the facial artery and vein. The facial artery is ligated away from the external carotid artery, so that in case the vessel retracts into the tissue it can be located and ligated and bleeding can be controlled. In case the ligature slips and the facial artery retracts; the posterior belly of digastric muscle is divided for easy location of the bleeding vessel.

The medial surface is related anteriorly to the mylohyoid muscle separated from it by the mylohyoid nerve and vessels and branches of the submental vessels. More posteriorly it is related to the styloglossus muscle, stylohyoid ligament and glossopharyngeal nerve which separate it from

Applied surgical anatomy 23

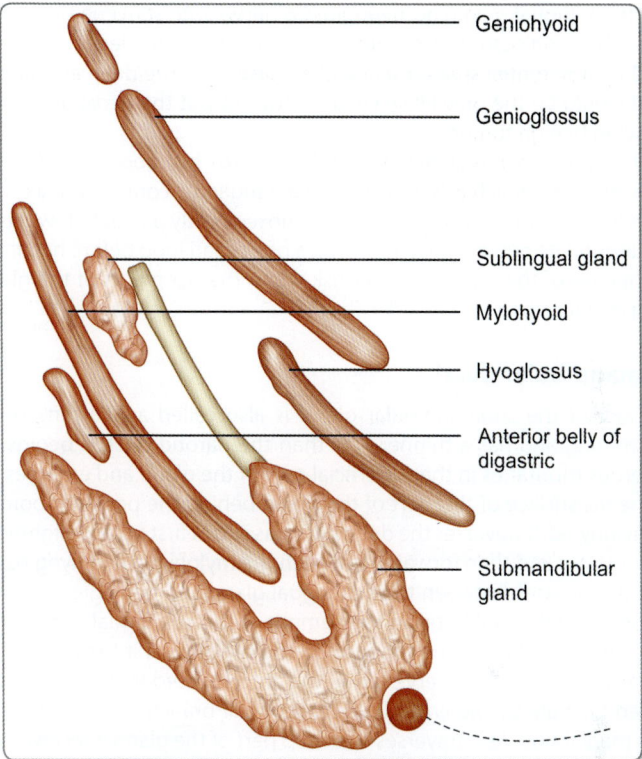

Figure 3.8 Relations of submandibular gland

the pharynx. In its intermediate part it is related to the styloglossus, lingual nerve, submandibular ganglion, hypoglossal nerve and deep lingual vein. The medial surface is related to the stylohyoid and posterior belly of digastric inferiorly. Anteriorly it is related to the anterior belly of digastric muscle and posteriorly it is related to stylohyoid and posterior belly of digastric muscles and parotid gland.

Relations of the deep part[4,12] (Figure 3.8)

Anteriorly sublingual gland is present and posteriorly it is related to stylohyoid muscle, posterior belly of digastric muscle and parotid gland.

Laterally it is related to mylohyoid muscle and superficial part of the gland and medially it is related to hyoglossus and styloglossus muscles.

Superiorly lingual nerve, submandibular ganglion and mucosa of the floor of mouth are present and inferiorly it is related to hypoglossal nerve and deep lingual vein. The hypoglossal nerve with its venae comitantes lies on the hyoglossus muscle but is separated from the deep aspect of the gland by a potential space. Escape of disease from the deep aspect of the gland would be the only likely circumstance to put the nerve at risk when removing benign tumors.

The lingual nerve arches gently downwards just above the deep part of the gland to which it is attached by a ganglionic connection, alongside which is a small blood vessel. The nerve subsequently passes below the duct then around its outer aspect in the form of a broad loop before heading for the mucosa of the tongue. It is at risk when the deep part of the gland is being mobilized.

Submandibular duct[4]

The duct of the submandibular gland is also called as Warton's duct. It is 5 cm long and has a thinner wall than the parotid duct. It begins from numerous tributaries in the superficial part of the gland and emerges from the medial surface of this part of the gland behind the posterior border of the mylohyoid. It traverses the deep part, passing at first up and slightly back for 4 or 5 mm and then forwards between the mylohyoid and hyoglossus.

It then passes between the sublingual gland and genioglossus muscle and opens in the oral floor on the summit of the sublingual papilla at the side of the frenulum of the tongue. On the hyoglossus it lies between the lingual and hypoglossal nerve but at the anterior border of the muscle it is crossed laterally by the lingual nerve, terminal branches of which ascend on its medial side. As it traverses the deep part of the gland it receives small tributaries draining this part of the gland.

The duct of the submandibular gland is longer and has a tortous, uphill course. Thus the secretions have to be emptied against gravity and there are increased chances of retention. Also, the mineral content of the secretion is high, especially calcium content which along with increased retention of secretions result into higher incidence of calculus formation and inflammatory pathologies.

Blood supply, lymphatics and nerve supply[12]

Branches of the facial and lingual arteries supply the submandibular gland and the corresponding veins drain it.

The lymph vessels drain into the submandibular and deep cervical lymph nodes.

Parasympathetic secretomotor supply is from the superior salivary nucleus of the facial nerve. The nerve fibers pass to the submandibular ganglion and other small ganglia close to the duct via the chorda tympani nerve and the lingual nerve. Postganglionic parasympathetic fibers reach the gland either directly or along the duct. Postganglionic sympathetic fibers reach the gland as a plexus of nerves around the facial and lingual arteries.

Sublingual glands

They are the smallest of the major salivary glands. They lie beneath the mucosa of the floor of the mouth causing an elevation, salivary eminence, on the floor of the oral cavity. Both the glands are in contact with the sublingual fossa on the lingual aspect of the mandible, close to the symphysis. They are mixed glands, but predominantly mucous. The gland is narrow, flat, shaped like an almond and weighs 3–4 gm.[12] The sublingual gland has an anterior and posterior segment.[7a]

Relations of the gland[12] (Figure 3.9)

Superiorly it is related to the mucosa of the floor of the oral cavity which is elevated by the gland to form sublingual fold. Inferiorly the gland is supported by the mylohyoid muscle.

Anteriorly it meets the gland of the opposite side at the midline, whereas posteriorly it is related to the deep part of the submandibular gland.

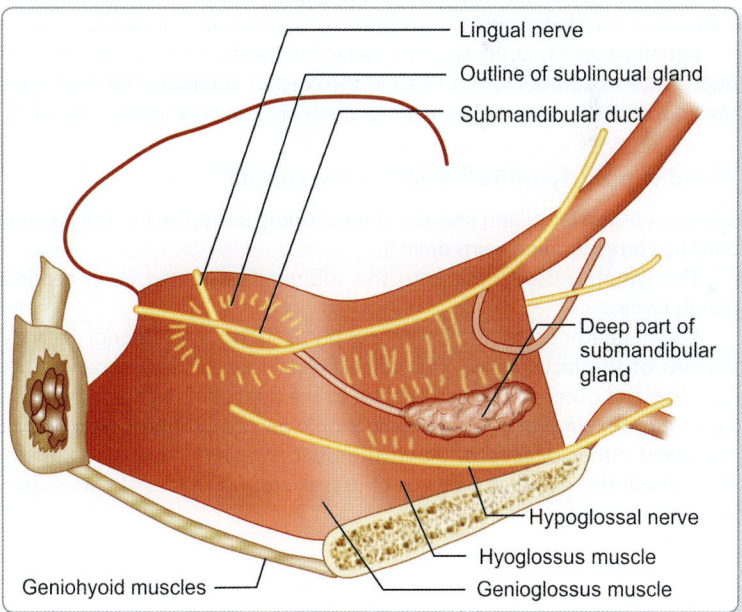

Figure 3.9 Superficial relations of submandibular gland

Medially, genioglossus muscle is present and is separated from the sublingual gland by lingual nerve and submandibular duct. Laterally, it is related to the sublingual fossa of the medial surface of the mandible.

Ducts of the gland

The anterior segment drains in the Bartholins duct which opens in the floor of the mouth or occasionally into very anterior sub-mandibular duct. The posteror segment drains into multiple ducts in the floor of mouth as well as ducts of Rivinus, which may enter into submandibular duct in the posterior floor of the mouth.[7a] There are 8–20 ducts of the sublingual gland. Of the smaller ducts most open separately on the summit of the sublingual fold and a few into submandibular duct. From anterior part of the gland, small rami arise from the major salivary duct and known as Bartholin's duct.[6]

The secretions of the sublingual glands are thick and mucoid in nature. The excretory ducts of the sublingual glands are very superficially located and open in the floor of mouth which is situated at a superior level than the gland. Hence, they easily get damaged and any trauma or infection of the ducts leads to salivary retention and formation of a mucous retention cyst which is called 'Ranula' due to its bluish color resembling the belly of a frog. Smaller or minor sublingual glands may be subdivided into two groups. Glands of one group send their ducts into adjacent submandibular duct and sometimes fused with anterior extension of submandibular gland.

Other group lies at the superior surface of the gland. They release short ducts 5–15 in number which open at the crest of sublingual eminence on the floor of the oral cavity. These minor ducts are known as ducts of Rivinus.[6]

Blood supply, lymphatics and nerve supply[12]

Branches of the facial and lingual arteries supply the submandibular gland and the corresponding veins drain it.

The lymph vessels drain into the submandibular and deep cervical lymph nodes.

Parasympathetic secretomotor supply is from the superior salivary nucleus of the facial nerve. The nerve fibers pass to the submandibular ganglion and other small ganglia close to the duct via the chorda tympani nerve and the lingual nerve. Postganglionic parasympathetic fibers reach the gland either directly or along the duct. Postganglionic sympathetic fibers reach the gland as a plexus of nerves around the facial and lingual arteries.

References

1. Standring S, Berkovitz BKB, Ruskell GL. Gray's Anatomy, Churchill Livingstone, Spain 1999;39(8):1290-8.
2. Bradley PJ. Pathology and treatment of salivary gland conditions. Surgery. 2006; 24(9):304-11.
3. DuBrul EL. The oral viscera. Sicher and DuBrul's Oral Anatomy. Ishiyaku EuroAmerica, Inc. St, louis. 1988;8(6):161-78.
3a. Saunders PR, Macpherson DW. Acute suppurative parotitis: A forgotten cause of upper airway obstruction. Oral Surg Oral Med Oral Pathol. 1991; 72:412-4.
4. Hollinshead WH. The Face. Anatomy for Surgeons: Vol I. The Head and Neck, Harper and Row Publishers, Philadelphia. 1982;6(9):291-324.
5. Cawson R, Gleeson M. Anatomy and physiology of the salivary glands. Gleeson M (Ed). Scott-Brown's Otolaryngology. Basic sciences, Butterworth Heinemann. Great Britian 1997;6(9):1/9/1-1/9/18.
6. Katz AD, Catalano P. The clinical significance of the various anastomotic branches of the facial nerve. Archives of Otolaryngol – Head and Neck Surg. 1987;113:959-62.
7. Snell RS. The Head and Neck. Clinical Anatomy, Lippincott Williams and Wilkins, Philadelphia. 2004;7(11):719-922.
7a. Williams MF. Sialolithiasis. Rice DH, Eisele DW, Editors. Salivary gland disorders. Otolaryngol Clin N Am. 1999;32(5):819-34.
8. Russel RCG, Williams NS, Bulstrode CJK. Bailey and Love's Short practice of surgery, Oxford University Press, New York. 2004;24.
9. Rankow RM, Polayes IM. Surgical anatomy and diagnosis. Diseases of Salivary glands. WB Saunders, Philadelphia. 1976;7:156-84.
10. John Hibbert. Scott-Brown's Laryngology and Head and Neck Surgery, Butterworth Heinemann, Great Britian. 1997;6(5),20:5/20/2.
11. McGregor IA, McGregor FM. Salivary glands. Cancer of the Face and Mouth. Pathology and management for surgeons, Churchill Livingstone. Edinburgh. 1986;25:569-606.
12. Bell RB, Dierks EJ, Homer L, Potter BE. Management and outcome of patients with malignant salivary gland tumors. J Oral Maxillofac Surg. 2005;63:917-28.
13. Strome M. The Parotid Neoplasm. Editor Pensak ML. Controversies in Otolaryngology. Publication Thieme. New York. 2001;22(65):344-7.
14. Hanna EY, Suen JY. The Parotid Neoplasm. Pensak ML (Ed). Controversies in Otolaryngology. Publication Thieme. New York 2001;22(66):348-54.
15. Wetmore SJ. Surgical landmarks for the facial nerve. Otolaryngol Clin North Am. 1991;24(3):505-30.
16. Conley JJ. Search for and identification of the facial nerve. Laryngoscope. 1978;88:172-5.

17. Pather N, Osman M. Landmark of Facial nerve: Implication for Parotidectomy. Surgical and Radiological Anatomy. 2006;28(2):170-5.
18. Pia F, Poliocarpo M, Dosdegani R, Olina M, Brovelli F, Aluffi P. Centripetal approach to the facial nerve in Parotid surgery: personal experience. Acta Otorhinolaryngol Ital. 2003;23:111-5.
19. Witt RL. Facial nerve function after partial superficial parotidectomy: an 11 years review 1987-97. Otolaryngol Head Neck Surg. 1999;121:210-3.
20. Farrior JB, Santini H. Facial nerve identification in children. Otolaryngol Head Neck Surg. 1985;93:173.

Historical perspective

chapter 4

The ancient Greeks referred to the parotid glands as para-auricular swellings. The historical development of knowledge of anatomy can be divided into early period from fifth century BC to early seventeenth century AD and a second salivary period from seventeenth century onwards.[1]

During the salivary period, maximum discovery of the salivary glands was done during 1634–1666. Marcello Malpighi gave the first definitive documentation summarizing all knowledge about the salivary glands from ancient times to the seventeenth century.[1]

Diseases of the salivary glands, and particularly the parotid, were recognized by Hippocrates (460–370 BC), and in the translation by Littre (1861) there are multiple references to suppurative and non-suppurative parotitis and the distinction between the former and that occurring in mumps. Paulus Aegineta (AD 607–690) makes but passing reference to parotitis as an affection of the glands about the ears, invoking the humoral theory.[2]

Abulcasis Al Zahrawi, AD 936–1013, from the western Caliphate, considered as Islam's greatest medieval surgeon, differentiated between malignancy of the floor of mouth and ranula, which he likened to a 'small frog', and advised incision and drainage.[2]

Thomas Wharton (1614–1673) had described the submandibular duct whereas Niels Steenson or Nicolaus Stenonis (1638–1686) had discovered the parotid duct on 7th April, 1660 during dissection and passed a silver probe into the animal's mouth from the parotid. Caspar Bartholin (1655–1738) has his name associated with the sublingual gland ducts as well as with the vulvo-vaginal glands. However the sublingual gland ducts are most commonly called ducts of Rivinus due to significant contribution from Auguste Quirini Rivini in this field.[2]

Andreas Vesalius (1514–1564) described the parotid gland whereas William Cheselden (1740) described the major salivary glands and also the parotid fistula. In 1561, Pierre Franco described tumors of the parotid gland as well as parotitis.[2]

Sebaceous glands were first described in four patients by Hamperl in a review of salivary glands from eighty-five subjects, in 1931.[3]

Prior to 18th century, salivary gland surgery progressed with glacial slowness. Major abscess or apostumes were poulticed and drained, but a salivary calculus was rarely extracted through the mouth. John Hunter resected a parotid tumor in 1785.[2]

Early parotidectomy was carried out in Ireland by Carmichael in 1818. He described a large tumor of the parotid gland which was present for 14 years. He performed the surgery on 14th December 1817 and was assisted by Todd and Colles.

McClellan is known to have performed at least 11 total parotidectomies. He performed the first parotidectomy on 14th May 1805 on Elizabeth McKee for a cancerous parotid.

Thomas Cawardine was the first to suggest that the facial nerve should be identified. According to Kidd, he was the first to have performed a parotidectomy with preservation of the facial nerve. Barbat has reported one single case in 1916. WE Sistrunk later suggested that its ramus marginalis branch be located first. Vilray Papin Blair also stressed the identification and preservation of the facial nerve. Ochsner and Adson and Ott endorsed facial nerve preservation. Adson and Ott are credited with describing a satisfactory technique of parotidectomy. Similarly noteworthy contributions have been made by Bailey, Janes, Furstenburg, State and many others.

McEvedy, in 1934, suggested the use of radiotherapy. In the first half of the 20th century surgeons frequently performed enucleation of the mixed tumor and used a standard 'T' shaped incision. Recurrence rates were high.

It was only after McFarland highlighted the drawback, that parotidectomy either superficial or total with facial nerve preservation for benign tumors was advocated by Janes (1940), Bailey (1941), Martin (1952) and Patey (1954).[4]

References

1. Pellegrini V M, Polayes IM. Historical background. Surgical Management. Diseases of Salivary glands. WB Saunders, Philadelphia. 1976;1:1-16.
2. Norman JE, McGurk M. History of salivary glands and mixed parotid tumor. Colour atlas and text of salivary glands - diseases, disorders and surgery. Mosby-Wolfe Spain. 1995;1:1.
3. Auclair PL, Ellis GL, Douglas GR. Other benign epithelial neoplasms. Ellis GL, Editor. Surgical pathology of the salivary glands. WB Saunders, Philadelphia. 1991;15:252-68.
4. Papadogeorgakis N, Chris A. Skouteris, Anastassios I. Mylonas, Angelos P, Angelopoulos. Superficial parotidectomy: technical modifications based on tumor characteristics. J Cranio Maxillofacs Surg. 2004;32:350-3.

chapter 5
Classifications

General classification of salivary gland diseases[1]
1. Developmental
    a. Aplasia – absence of gland
    b. Atresia – absence of duct
    c. Aberrancy – ectopic gland
2. Enlargement of gland
    a. Inflammatory
        i. Viral: Mumps, Coxsackie-A, CMV, Influenza, Para-influenza virus
        ii. Bacterial
        iii. Allergic
        iv. Sarcoidosis
        v. Obstructive
    b. Non-inflammatory
        i. Autoimmune: Sjögren's syndrome, Mickulicz's disease
        ii. Alcoholic cirrhosis
        iii. Diabetes mellitus
        iv. Nutritional deficiency
        v. HIV associated
3. Cysts
    a. Extravasation cysts
    b. Retention cysts
    c. Ranula
4. Tumors of salivary glands
    a. Benign
    b. Malignant
5. Necrotizing sialometaplasia
6. Salivary gland dysfunction
    a. Sialorrhea
    b. Xerostomia

Many researchers have given numerous classifications for salivary gland tumors. However, the most recent and most accepted classification is as follows:

WHO histological classification of tumors of the salivary gland, 2002[2]

- Malignant epithelial tumors:
  - Acinic cell carcinoma — 8550/3
  - Mucoepidermoid carcinoma — 8430/3
  - Adenoid cystic carcinoma — 8200/3
  - Polymorphous low-grade adenocarcinoma — 8525/3
  - Epithelial – myoepithelial carcinoma — 8562/3
  - Clear cell carcinoma, not otherwise specified — 8310/3
  - Basal cell adenocarcinoma — 8147/3
  - Sebaceous carcinoma — 8410/3
  - Sebaceous lymphadenocarcinoma — 8410/3
  - Cystadenocarcinoma — 8440/3
  - Low-grade cribriform adenocarcinoma
  - Mucinous adenocarcinoma — 8480/3
  - Oncocytic carcinoma — 8290/3
  - Salivary duct carcinoma — 8500/3
  - Adenocarcinoma, not otherwise specified — 8140/3
  - Myoepithelial carcinoma — 8982/3
  - Carcinoma ex pleomorphic adenoma — 8941/3
  - Carcinosarcoma — 8980/3
  - Metastasizing pleomorphic adenoma — 8940/1
  - Squamous cell carcinoma — 8070/3
  - Small cell carcinoma — 8041/3
  - Large cell carcinoma — 8012/3
  - Lymphoepithelial carcinoma — 8082/3
  - Sialoblastoma — 8974/1
- Benign epithelial tumors:
  - Pleomorphic adenoma — 8940/0
  - Myoepithelioma — 8982/0
  - Basal cell adenoma — 8147/0
  - Warthin tumor — 8561/0
  - Oncocytoma — 8290/0
  - Canalicular adenoma — 8149/0
  - Sebaceous adenoma — 8410/0
  - Lymphadenoma
    - Sebaceous — 8410/0
    - Non-sebaceous — 8410/0
  - Ductal papillomas
    - Inverted ductal papilloma — 8503/0
    - Intraductal papilloma — 8503/0
    - Sialadenoma papilleferum — 8406/0
  - Cystadenoma — 8440/0

- Soft tissue tumors
  - Hemangioma   9120/0
- Hematolymphoid tumors
  - Hodgkin lymphoma
  - Diffuse large B-cell lymphoma   9680/3
  - Extranodal marginal zone B-cell lymphoma   9699/3
- Secondary tumors

Based on morphology code of the International Classification of Diseases for Oncology ICD-O, 821 and the Systematized Nomenclature of Medicine.

Behavior is coded as follows:
0- benign tumors
1-borderline or uncertain behavior
3-malignant tumors

References

1. WHO manual of classification of diseases 2003.
2. Auclair PL, Ellis GL, Douglas GR, Wenig BM, Janney CG. Salivary gland neoplasms: General considerations. Ellis GL (Ed). Surgical pathology of the salivary glands. WB Saunders, Philadelphia. 1991;9:135-64.

Diagnosis and diagnostic aids

chapter 6

In salivary gland disease a careful history and examination will usually provide a correct diagnosis, but the major salivary glands may pose a diagnostic challenge because not only are they affected by specific local pathology but also by systemic disease. Conditions affecting adjacent structures, bone, muscle connective tissue and lymph nodes may masquerade as a salivary gland swelling.

History

A meticulous history leads to the determination of the nature of the lesion in the salivary glands. It must include:

1. *Onset:* The nature of onset of the growth is often significant. If the onset is painless, gradual but continuous a tumor is suggested. However, if it is sudden and painful, it is suggestive of an inflammatory pathology, although rapidly growing tumor with overlying infection may mimic the same situation.
2. *Duration:* An old lesion with a history of slow, steady growth is usually benign or low grade malignant tumor. If an old lesion has a history of remission and exacerbation associated with pain, it is most often inflammatory. A new lesion without pain which grows rapidly is suggestive of early malignancy.
3. *Progress and rapidity of growth:* A malignant tumor grows rapidly whereas a benign tumor grows slowly and steadily. The benign tumor might attain large size with only pressure symptoms, whereas the malignant tumor infiltrates the surrounding vital structures and may cause pain. A tumor never regresses, although there might be a period of quiescence.
4. *Extent of the growth:* A benign tumor might attain a huge size and produce only a cosmetic defect but a malignant tumor will produce functional deficit as well if it invades adjacent structures. The extent of the growth must be recorded in all three dimensions to gauge the degree of involvement of surrounding structures. In addition it helps to know the surgical defect that will be created. Ultrasound, CT scans, MRI scans are of immense help in knowing the extent of the growth.
5. *Symptoms associated with the growth:* Pain suggests inflamma-tion or secondary infection. Paresthesia, tingling and numbness, weakness of

muscles supplied by the nerve may be suggestive of infiltration of the nerve by tumor cells. Salivary gland tumors most commonly present as an asymptomatic mass. Pain is not a reliable indicator of malignancy. Cystic enlargement, hemorrhage, or infection can cause pain in benign tumors. Malignant tumors often enlarge without symptoms, but when pain occurs, it is often the result of neural involvement and carries a worse prognosis. If nasal obstruction is also present, the clinician should suspect a tumor in the nasal or paranasal sinuses, possibly arising from a minor salivary gland.
6. *Coincidental conditions:* Sometimes salivary gland tumors may be associated with other conditions. Breast cancer is associated with a high-risk of parotid tumors.[1,2]
7. *Secretions:* Secretions if purulent may suggest an infective pathology.

Physical examination

Inspection and palpation are most important diagnostically. Any palpable enlargement is abnormal. Generally, the neoplasms originate as firm, smooth, rounded nodules that vary in size depending upon their duration. A history of sudden growth or ulceration usually suggests malignancy.

The major salivary glands are palpated, and the orifices of the ducts are observed for saliva output. Normally, clear saliva should be expressed when the gland is pressed and "milked." Both parotid and submandibular lymph nodes may appear as swellings appearing primarily in the glands. Bimanual palpation of these lesions placing one finger intraorally and one extraorally must be done to locate and trace the extent of the growth. Mobility denotes that the lesion has not infiltrated the surrounding tissues. A malignant tumor and its lymphatic spread except early lymph node metastases are not readily movable. If the tumor is fluctuant, the tumor probably is cystic.

However, regardless of the sites both benign and malignant tumors resemble each other clinically. Histopathology is the only solution to diagnosis.

Parotid tumors

The diagnosis of parotid gland tumors usually does not pose a significant difficulty. The patient presents with a complaint of an asymptomatic mass noted during shaving or washing of the face. Many patients do present with a small incision overlying the lesion, wherein a previous misdiagnosis of sebaceous cyst was made. The sebaceous cyst moves with the skin movement but a benign tumor remains fixed on movement of the skin. The transverse process of the axis, in cases of asymmetry of the process,

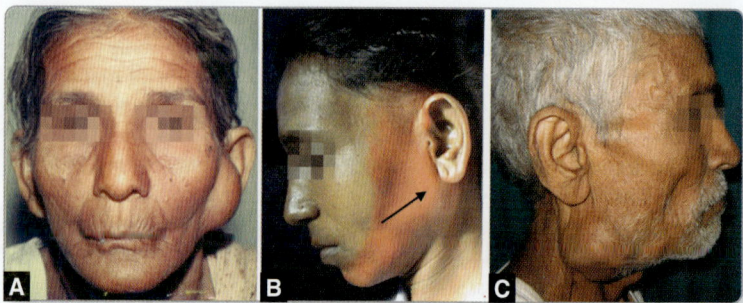

Figures 6.1A to C (A) Parotid neoplasm involving the superficial lobe. (Note the typical location); (B) Early benign tumor of parotid not showing raising of ear lobule; (C) Multi-lobulated tumor of tail of parotid

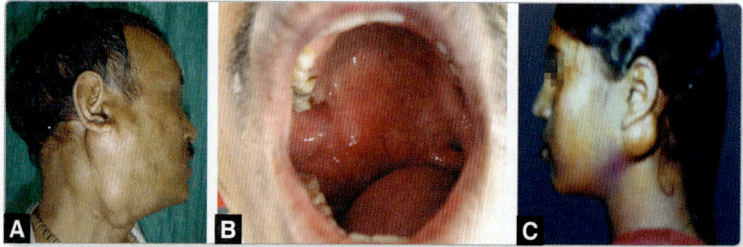

Figures 6.2A to C (A) Multilobulated parotid tumor with deep lobe involvement; (B) Showing deviation of soft palate to opposite side; (C) Typical parotid tumor with raising of ear lobule

was also mistaken for parotid neoplasm before the advent of computerized scanning.[3] Tumors of the parotid gland will typically present as solitary painless mobile masses, most often located at the tail of the gland. As the superficial lobe tumors grow in size, the lobule of the ear gets raised. Deep lobe neoplasms are more difficult to diagnose and can be obscure for many years until they are diagnosed on routine oral examinations, due to medial displacement of the oropharyngeal wall. Malignant neoplasms of the deep lobe may present with Eustachian tube obstruction and pain. A diagnosis cannot be reached until a CT scan or MRI scan is obtained. It could be misdiagnosed as temporomandibular joint syndrome. Hence bizarre complaints involving referred pain to the ear and lateral aspect of the ramus of mandible or TMJ should be investigated using radiological techniques.

It is important to document function of the facial nerve when evaluating parotid tumors, because the nerve runs through the gland, and evidence of decreased motor function of the nerve thus has diagnostic significance.

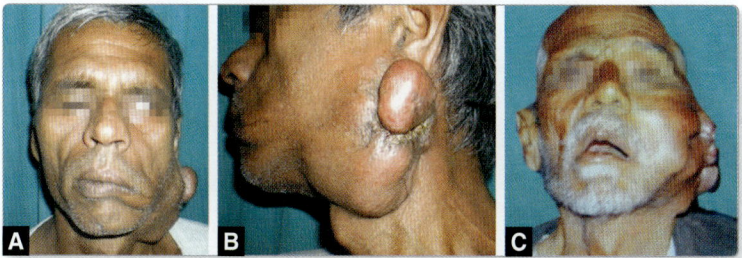

Figures 6.3A to C (A) Malignant parotid tumor with facial nerve paralysis. Note: Drooping of corner of mouth and bells sign; (B) Involvement of overlying skin is also suggestive of malignant tumor; (C) Malignant parotid tumor with fungation

Facial nerve paralysis (Bell's palsy) is usually indicative of malignancy. Rarely, benign tumors may cause paralysis by either sudden rapid growth or the presence of an infection. Other findings suggesting malignancy include multiple masses, a fixed mass with invasion of surrounding tissue, and the presence of cervical lymphadenopathy.

Submandibular gland tumors

The submandibular triangle masses usually present as inflammatory swellings but a neoplasm must always be considered in the differential diagnosis of the submandibular mass. The most important reason for such a consideration is that a neoplasm can also cause obstruction of the gland and present with inflammatory symptoms. The most important symptoms going in favor of an obstructive pathology are increased pain and tenderness associated with meals. In addition the calculus can also be located by bimanual palpation of the gland and by radiological investigations.

A submandibular gland tumor presents as an asymptomatic mass or lump in the neck inferior to the lower border of the mandible. Bimanual palpation, with one hand intraorally on the floor of the mouth and the other extraorally below the mandible, is necessary to evaluate the glands adequately.

It is important to check for the dysfunction of the cranial nerves related to the submandibular triangle viz marginal mandibular branch of the facial nerve, lingual and mental branches of the mandibular division of the trigeminal nerve and presence of lymphadenopathy of the jugular chain of lymph nodes. Fixity of the mass to the mandible and overlying skin should also be noted. Marginal mandibular nerve weakness is not a conclusive diagnostic criterion for malignancy of the submandibular gland because it is also seen in sarcoid as a variant of Heerfordt's syndrome.

38 Salivary gland pathologies

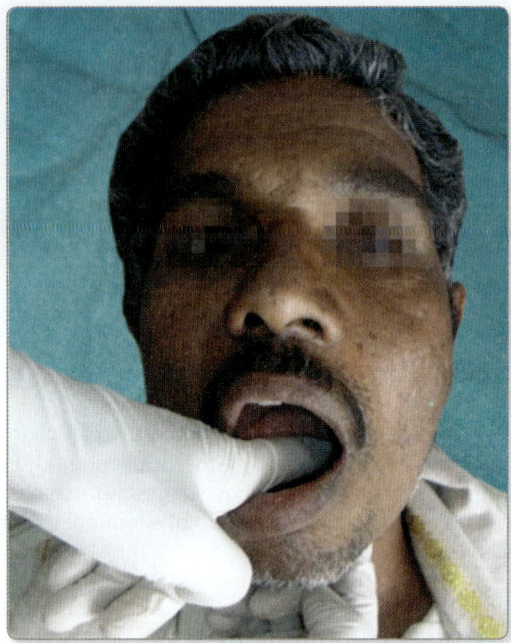

Figure 6.4 Bimanual palpation of submandibular gland

Sublingual salivary gland

Sublingual salivary gland lies in the floor of the mouth between the mylohyoid muscle and the submandibular duct. It lies in close relation to the lingual vessels and the nerve and the hypoglossal nerve. A sublingual gland tumor presents as a mass in the floor of the mouth often displacing the tongue. Due to its proximity to the floor of the mouth, a malignant tumor affecting the submandibular gland ulcerates the floor of the mouth quite early in its course.

Minor salivary glands

An intraoral accessory gland tumor presents as a prominent, asymptomatic swelling and is often mistaken for a fibroma or an abscess. Tumors of the minor salivary glands are usually smooth masses located on the hard or soft palate. Ulceration of the overlying mucosa should raise suspicion of malignancy. They are evaluated invasion of associated structures.

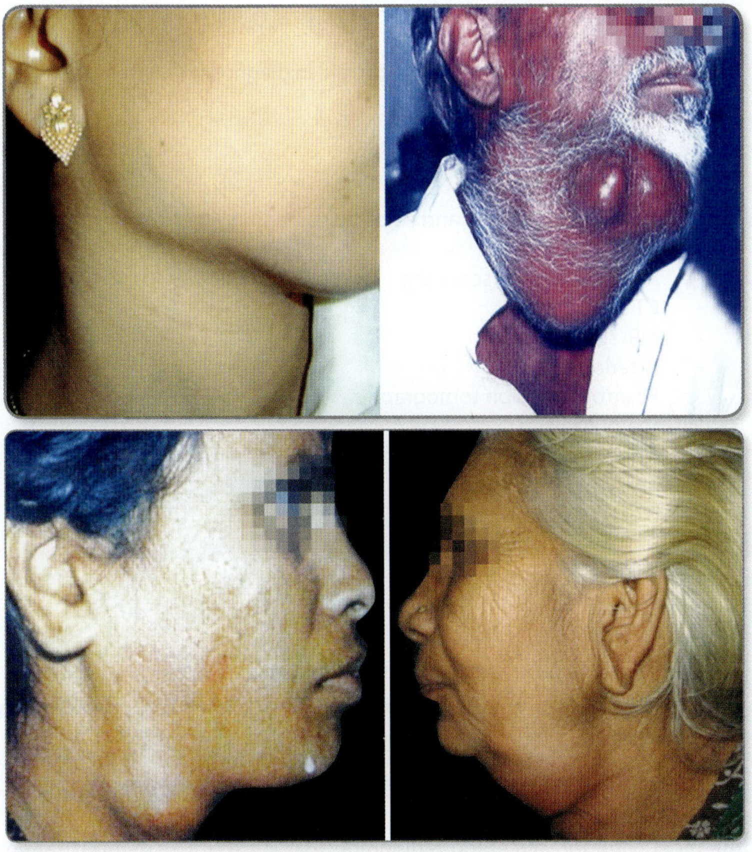

Diagnosis and diagnostic aids 39

Figure 6.5 Varied presentations of submandibular gland tumors

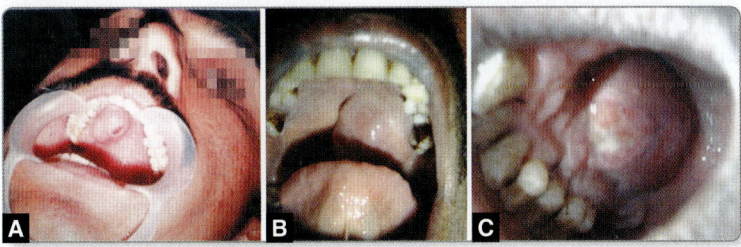

Figures 6.6A to C (A, B) Pleomorphic adenoma of palatal minor salivary glands; (C) Malignant tumor of palatal salivary gland

Diagnostic aids

Investigations that can be performed to aid in diagnosing the salivary gland neoplasms are as follows:
1. Diagnostic imaging:
   - Routine radiographs
   - Ultrasonography
   - Doppler ultrasound and color-flow imaging
   - Sialography
   - Radionucleotide scanning
   - CT scan
   - MRI scan
   - Arteriography
   - Positron emission tomography
2. Histopathology:
   - Fine needle aspiration cytopathology
   - Incisional biopsy
   - Frozen sections

Diagnostic imaging

Plain radiographs

Plain radiographs have been used for many years to visualize calcification within the glands and demonstrate bony changes in the adjacent structures. In addition they are used to show the distant effects of salivary gland metastases. Extraoral views which can be used include AP, Frontal view, lateral view, lateral oblique, orthopantomogram (OPG) and intraoral views include occlusal, intraoral periapical view (IOPA). OPG is the most common screening radiograph that is used. The demonstration of parenchymal calcification, and in particular where there are a number of well-defined opacities, it may be almost pathognomonic of a cavernous-type hemangioma. The plain radiograph is an insensitive method to show calcification as compared with CT scans. Calcification which may be projected over salivary glands, mimicking glandular calcification, includes tonsiloliths and calcification of cervical lymph nodes or laryngeal cartilages. Demonstration of invasive change in adjacent bony structures by plain radiographs usually underestimates the extent of the disease because at least 30% of mineral content of the bone must be lost before it appears on the radiograph. Salivary gland enlargements are not seen on plain radiographs. CT scans and MRI imaging have a demonstrable edge over plain radiography in this respect. In addition plain radiographs can show metastatic disease in distant tissues. Major utility of plain radiography is to demonstrate sialolith and calcification of salivary gland parenchyma. A cheek blow-out AP view is used to identify any sialoloith in the parotid duct.

Diagnosis and diagnostic aids 41

Ultrasonography

Ultrasonography applied to diagnosis of salivary gland diseases involve transmission of sound energy into salivary tissues, which is attenuated as it passes through tissues depending on the acoustic properties of the tissue and receiving that energy after it has been reflected by the tissues and recording it so that it can be presented for our interpretation.[4,5] Ultrasound has a considerable potential as a method of clinical investigation of the salivary glands as it is noninvasive, utilizes non-ionizing radiation, gives good soft tissue discrimination, has excellent sensitivity for mass lesions and can be repeated as frequently as required. It helps to distinguish a cystic lesion from a solid mass in space occupying lesion. Normal salivary gland is homogenously relatively hyperechogenic on USG than adjacent muscle. Tumors and cysts are more hypoechoic than normal parenchyma. It is a more sensitive scan than CT for identification of small lesions less than 1 cm in diameter.[6] Neoplasms appear as solid masses. A relatively well defined capsule with a homogenous central area is indicative of a benign or low-grade malignant tumor. An irregular or ill-defined capsule with complicated heterogenous center indicates malignant or inflammatory

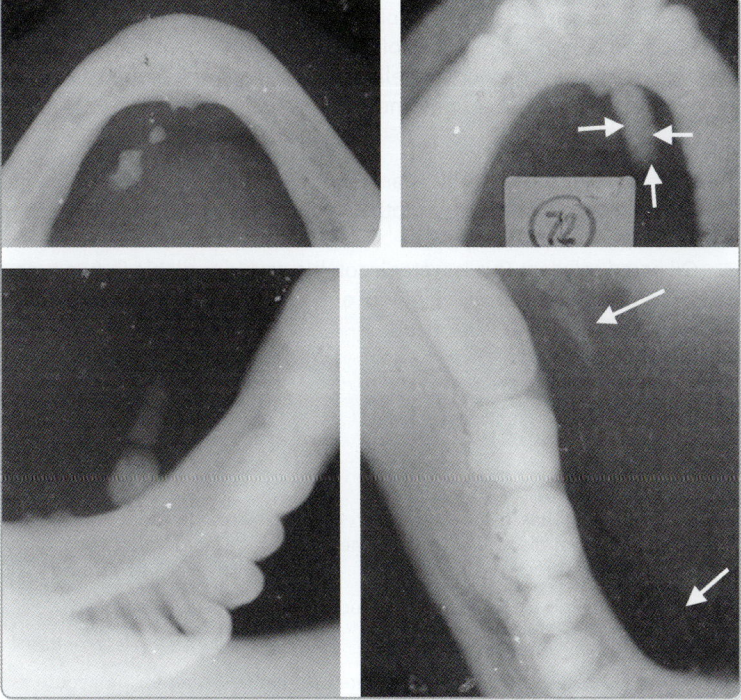

Figure 6.7 Occlusal radiograhs showing radiopaque calculus in Whartons duct

changes. Adenolymphoma shows the appearance of predominantly cystic lesion, with well-defined internal septa whereas Pleomorphic adenoma shows small buds presenting in the capsule, which might not be a constant finding. Overall sensitivity of USG in detecting parotid tumors is very high. The drawbacks of USG include its inability demonstrate the facial nerve in relation to the parotid gland and to define the extent of tumors extending outside the deep surface or of extraglandular lesions such as nasopharyngeal tumors invading the deep aspect of the gland. In addition, it is difficult to image the deep lobes of the major salivary glands.[4]

Doppler ultrasound and color-flow imaging

Doppler ultrasound and color-flow imaging enables immediate recognition of vascular structures. It allows confident discrimination between small vessels and ducts and rapid assessment of the vascularity of the mass lesions. It is particularly useful in showing the presence or absence of vascular flow within low signal lesions which allows distinction between cystic lesions with thick contents and some solid tumors with low signal central portions.

Sialography

Sialography is a specialized radiological technique which involves the intubation of the principal duct of the salivary gland and instillation of radiopaque contrast medium to delineate the ductal system and any other spaces in continuity. The contrast mediums used are iodine based solutions.

They are classified as follows:
1. *Ionic aqueous solution:* This is an aqueous (water soluble) solution and is available in two types, viz Iothalamate (Conray 480) and Metrizoate (Triosil)
2. *Oil based solution:* This is water insoluble and is available in two types: Iodized poppy seed oil – Lipiodol and Water insoluble organic iodine compounds such as Pantopaque.

Dye type	Advantage	Disadvantage
Oil based	Densely radiopaque	Extravasated dye may remain in tissues for months
	Good contrast	Foreign body reaction
	High viscosity – slow excretion from gland – adequate time for the procedure	Requires increased pressure for introduction into duct – may force calculi deeper into the duct
Water based	Less viscosity – Easily introduced	Lesser medium is needed.
	Rapidly excreted	Less radiopaque – less contrast
	Easily absorbed and excreted if extravasated	Limited time for procedure as excreted fast

Diagnosis and diagnostic aids

Its chief value is in assessment of obstructive pathology. It has limited abilities to demonstrate intraglandular masses, which it does by primarily showing distortion of ductal system. Because of arborising nature of the ducts, any sizeable mass smaller than 1 cm in diameter will be shown. Neither is there any specificity about appearance of such lesions nor is there a predictive value for benign or malignant lesion. The impact of sialography in the management of mass lesions is restricted. It aids in determination of the tumor, its location, its origin (whether intrinsic or extrinsic), the presence of glandular impairment, and the suggestion of involvement of adjacent tissues. Centrally located lesion shows a characteristic appearance of ball-in-hand when a defect is located within the gland.

Indications for sialography
1. Obstructive pathologies like stricture, mucous plugs, hypocalcified calculi, external compressions.
2. Degenerative conditions.
3. Chronic inflammatory conditions (chronic sialodentis, sjögren's syndrome)
4. Intra and extra glandular tumors
5. Ductal anamolies (perforations, sialoceles, fistulas)

Contraindications for sialography
1. Allergy to the dye.
2. Acute inflammatory conditions. The injection of dye in acute inflammation will cause severe pain and can lead to necrosis of the gland.

Procedure
1. The orifice of the duct is identified and isolated.
2. Local anesthesia is infiltrated around the opening.
3. The duct opening is dilated by probing with a blunt probe like a lacrymal probe.
4. The duct is cannulated using a no. 22 canula and the canula is secured in place with a circumferential suture around the duct.

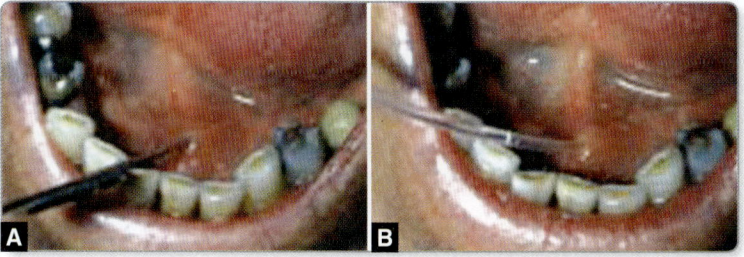

Figures 6.8A and B (A) Dilation of duct with lacrimal probe; (B) Cannulation of duct

5. The dye is loaded in a Leur lock syringe which is attached to the canula. The dye is slowly pushed, with simultaneously massaging the gland. The injection is continued until the patient feels discomfort due to pressure.
6. If the piston of the syringe is released the dye tends to flow back due to increased pressure in the gland. To prevent back flow of the dye the piston is held in place with the help of adhesive tape.
7. The X-rays are taken at regular interval as the die is filled (filling phase) and flows out of the duct.
8. The salivation is stimulated to empty the gland after the procedure.

Interpretation

1. The normal salivary gland shows a "tree in winter" or "leaf less tree" appearance for parotid gland and "bush in winter" appearance for submandibular gland, because in the functional gland the saliva present in the acini prevents the entry of the dye in them and thus, only the ductules and the ducts are seen.

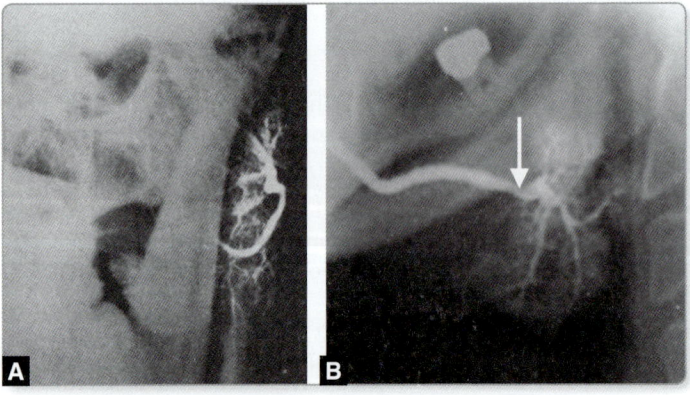

Figures 6.9A and B (A) Tree in winter appearance of normal parotid gland; (B) Bush in winter appearance of normal submandibular gland

2. In case of the chronic sialadenitis, the gland has the "leafy tree" or the "blossom tree appearance" as the non functional acini are empty and the eye enters in them and thus at the end of the ductules a round ball is seen.

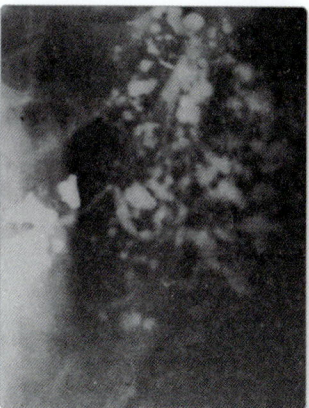

Figure 6.10 Blossom tree appearance

3. In case of Sjögren's syndrome and Mickulickz's disease, there is "snow storm" or "branchless fruit laden tree" appearance.

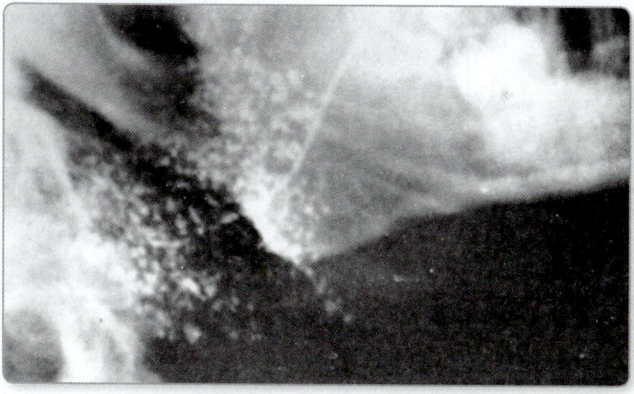

Figure 6.11 Branchless fruit laden tree appearance

4. When there is a stricture of mucous plug in the duct, a filling defect is seen. In case of multiple strictures a sausage string appearance is seen.
5. In case of perforation of the duct or sialocele the spillage of the dye in the soft tissue is seen.
6. In case of intra glandular tumors the normal glandular structure surrounds the tumor and thus a "cannon ball" appearance is produced.
7. The extra glandular tumor displaces the glandular structure is displaced to one side and produces a "ball in hand appearance".

46 Salivary gland pathologies

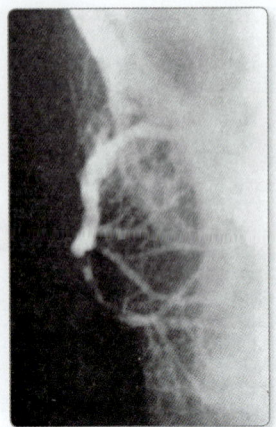

Figure 6.12 Ball in hand appearance

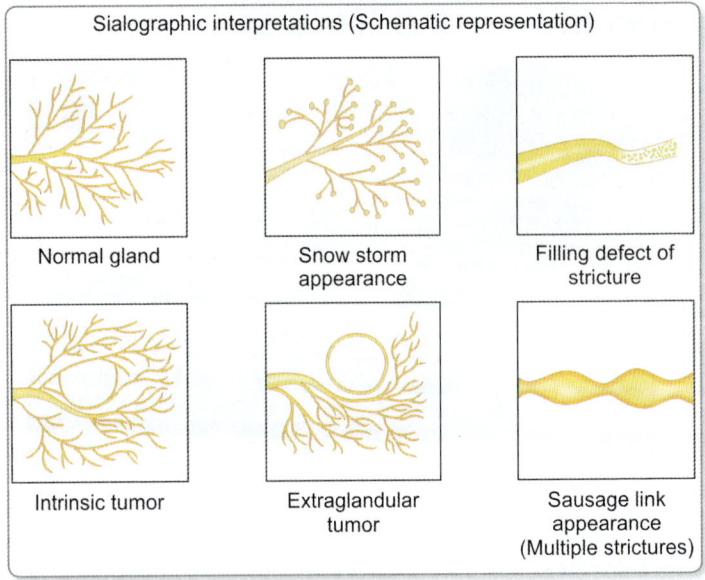

Figure 6.13 Schematic representation of various sialographic appearances

Radionucleotide scanning

Radionucleotide scanning is a valuable diagnostic tool in the evaluation of salivary gland physiology and pathology. It can be used in evaluating patients wherein for some or the other reason a sialogram is contraindicated. These scans are useful in differentiating between acute obstructive and non-obstructive sialoadenitis, showing presence of parenchymal masses greater than 1 cm in diameter and in few cases in identification of specific types of tumors.[7]

Static scanning
Imaging of the head and neck, usually with frontal projections is done 10–15 minutes after IV injection of 200 MBq technetium-99m pertechnetate. Tumors will be demonstrated if they are of a size above the resolution of the system, i.e. any mass more than 1.5 cm in diameter or larger. Space occupying lesions, as delineated by radioisotopic study are classified as hot, warm and cold lesions. The majority of tumors above this size, whether benign or malignant, show up as areas of decreased activity, or 'cold spots'. Major exceptions are Warthin's tumor[5] and certain lymphomas which concentrate isotope activity and appear as persistent 'hot spot'.[4] Carcinomas are thought to replace the normal glandular cells completely and appear as 'cold' lesions of decreased activity. Mixed tumors are composed of epithelial and stromal elements and may present a variable appearance depending on their histologic components. Most of the mixed tumors will appear as 'warm' lesions with an uptake similar to normal glandular tissue.[5] Apart from diagnosing secondary neoplasms which were not diagnosed prior to the investigation, static scans have no realistic effect on treatment planning.[4]

Dynamic scanning
It relies upon acquiring images throughout the scan. After the radionuclide is injected images are obtained initially at one minute intervals until end of scan. A dose of 50–100 MBq of technetium-99m pertechnetate is used. Computer generated graphs and digital images are used for assessment. The shape of the curve gives information of the function of the gland. Initial segment shows a fairly rapid rise (good ability to concentrate) followed by a sharp fall (normal excretion) in normal glands. If activity rises during excretion, it suggests duct obstruction but good ability to concentrate. If curve is relatively flat it suggests a gland with hampered ability to concentrate and excrete.

Nuclear imaging is an extremely sensitive method to show distant metastases, particularly in bone. This technique requires lesser radiation exposure of the patient than conventional radiography.

CT scan
CT scan images provide excellent soft tissue details that show not only the lesion but also involvement of the surrounding structures. It can be used to evaluate masses involving the parotid gland and adjacent structures and their relation to the facial nerve.

48 Salivary gland pathologies

On an axial CT scan, the relationship of the parotid mass to the facial nerve can be inferred by noting the relation to the retromandibular vein. Lateral displacement of the vein indicates a mass medial to the facial nerve whereas lack of or medial displacement may indicate a tumor superficial to the facial nerve.

The criteria of nerve involvement in parotid neoplasms on CT rely on bony changes along the course of the facial nerve which include bone erosion, sclerotic margins and widening of the normal diameter of the fallopian canal or stylomastoid foramen.[8]

MRI scan

MRI scan relies on electromagnetic properties of protons and in particular on the energy released when such particles decay from a higher to a relatively lower energy state within an externally applied magnetic field. MRI differs from CT in its apparent sensitivity to calcification. Heavily calcified tissue such as cortical bone or calculi produces no significant signal on MRI and is distinguished as a signal void. Thus dystrophic calcification of a tumor is not visible. The soft tissue contrast obtainable with MRI allows very good assessment of majority of the salivary masses. Benign or low-grade

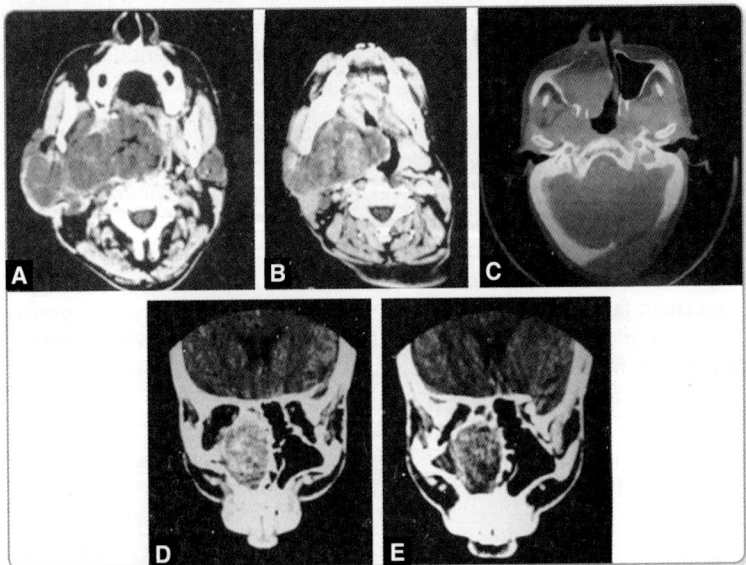

Figures 6.14A to E (A,B) Axial CT scan showing parotid tumor involving both lobes of parotid and extending up to skull base; (C) Axial CT scan showing minor salivary gland tumor involving the maxillary sinus and pterygoid plates; (D, E) Coronal CT scan showing involvement of posterior part of nasopharynx by tumor of palatal salivary gland

neoplasms have well-defined margins with relatively homogenous low signal intensity on T1-weighted images and high signal on T2-weighted images, which is thought to reflect high proportion of serous and mucinous products present. By contrast, high grade malignancies have poorly defined margins and tend to have heterogeneous low signal on both T1-and T2-weighted images, reflecting the high nuclear-cytoplasm ratio and lack of serous and mucinous material. Adenolymphoma has a relatively characteristic appearance as with ultrasound, possessing smooth margins but with a markedly heterogeneous central area and some peripheral signal aberrations which may be due to hemorrhage. Advantages of MRI are that, in case of parotid tumors, it can give the relation of the tumor to the retromandibular vein, carotid artery as well as facial nerve. However, a potential disadvantage of MRI as compared to CT scan is a relatively restricted field of view. A tumor might appear to be entirely intraglandular when it has already metastasized to cervical lymph nodes and many times may be outside the area imaged. Intravenous contrast agent viz gadolinium, assist in tumor delineation. The edge of the lesion may be better assessed following contrast and internal structure of the tumors is best seen in post-gadolinium images. Unsuspected infiltration of a malignancy can also be seen after contrast enhancement. The major criterion of malignancy is presence of ill-defined, infiltrating tumor margin but a smooth margin cannot rule out aggressive changes. It also helps in differentiation of post-operative fibrosis and recurrent tumor which demonstrate marked contrast uptake revealing the entire extent of the lesion.

Perineural spread can be diagnosed early on MRI due to better soft tissue delineation. The criteria of nerve involvement include replacement of normal perineural fat with tumor, enhancement with gadolinium (regardless of size) and increased size of the nerve in question (regardless of enhancement).[8] However, contrast MRI use is reserved only in suspected recurrence cases and to know the margins of a potentially malignant lesion.

Arteriography

Arteriography is important in the study of salivary gland tumors because it not only defines the vasculature of the tumor, but also delineates the origin of the vascular supply. This delineation can aid the surgeon in preoperative planning of the surgical procedure.

Positron emission tomography

Positron Emission Tomography scans have not gained wide application in the imaging of tumors of the salivary glands. The reasons for this are that salivary glands have a variable and inconsistent uptake of ^{18}F Fluorodeoxyglucose (FDG) which is a radiotracer most commonly used with PET scans. Hence ^{18}FDG-PET is unreliable both in tumor detection and in distinguishing benign from malignant tumors. In addition CT, MRI, clinical examination, have a high degree of accuracy. Also CT and MRI are high resolution studies which provide the anatomic details necessary for treatment planning that ^{18}FDG-PET fail to provide. Finally, the ^{18}FDG-PET is too expensive and is not cost effective. However ^{18}FDG-PET measures the metabolic activity in various tissues and hence is superior to CT and MRI in diagnosing recurrence and differentiating it from postoperative fibrosis. Since it can measure tumor metabolism, it can be used to evaluate tumor proliferation rates or tumor hypoxia that can be used to optimize treatment strategy such as fractionation scheme for radiotherapy or sequence for combined therapy. In a study, thirteen pleomorphic adenomas of the parotid gland were evaluated by computed tomography (CT), magnetic resonance imaging (MRI), Gallium scintigraphy, Technetium scintigraphy and FDG-positron emission tomography (PET). Pleomorphic adenomas were histologically classified into the following three types: epithelial, intermediate and mesenchymal, based on their dominant histological components. The accumulation of FDG did not differ significantly among the three types. Since the accumulation of FDG was significantly correlated with the tumor size, FDG-PET could reflect tumor growth ability more apparently than the other nuclear or imaging modalities.[9]

Histopathology

Fine needle aspiration cytopathology

Fine needle aspiration cytopathology as a diagnostic tool for salivary gland neoplasms has gained importance quite late after its inception in the Scandinavian countries in 1930's. This emergence is based on numerous studies that have demonstrated the high accuracy of fine needle aspiration in the diagnosis of salivary gland lesions. FNA of a parotid mass is controversial. If the diagnosis is benign, it is by no means absolute. On the other hand when a lesion is associated with physical findings such as nerve paralysis, very hard consistency, rapid growth or fixation to the deeper structures, FNA may be helpful in treatment planning. In a debilitated patient with a benign tumor and in a patient with a previous history of cancer (Lung / breast/ kidney) it may help in avoiding surgery. It may also yield a metastatic node which might change the treatment plan drastically.[10] According to most sources the diagnostic accuracy of FNA is 98% for benign tumors, 93% for malignant tumors and 88% for metastatic tumors. The diagnostic accuracy of FNA in addition to its cost containment and low associated morbidity rate makes it a much more feasible preoperative procedure for tumor assessment and directing subsequent therapy.[11] Salivary glands are easily accessible to needle aspiration. However, the risk of tumor dissemination or implantation is an important consideration because even if fine needles are used they will cause some degree of micro trauma during their passage into the tissues and increase the risk of local neoplastic spread along the needle tract and at distant sites through punctured blood and lymph vessels.[12] However with use of thinner guage needles for aspiration biopsy, implantation of tumor cells along the needle tract have not been reported. Arguments in support of FNA are cost containment, negligible associated morbidity and/or complications, rapidity in arriving at a diagnosis, high diagnostic accuracy and ability to use this procedure in determining patient management. However limitations of the aspirate are that limited histologic architectural features are seen and the tumor – stroma interface which is of importance in diagnosis of many salivary tumors can not be seen. Also, the status of invasion by the tumor, which is the most important criteria in predicting biologic behavior, is not disclosed by FNA. The sensitivity and specificity of FNA in salivary gland tumor diagnoses depends on the access to the cytopathologist who is both skilled and interested in the technique.[13] The overall sensitivity of FNAB of salivary gland ranges from 85.5 to 99% and the overall specificity ranges from 96.3 to 100%.[14] However, FNA of salivary gland lesions may be as reliable as frozen sections and pose a significantly lesser surgical risk than open biopsy. Koivuniemi et al have reported a false positive diagnostic rate of 2.3% and false negative rate of 5.5% with aspiration biopsy in salivary gland and other head and neck tumors.[11]

Incisional biopsy

Incisional biopsy is usually used to diagnose suspected systemic diseases. It is usually indicated when there is a soft enlargement of the salivary gland and is usually contraindicated if a firm, discrete mass indicative of a tumor is present.[14] A discrete salivary mass should never be subjected to incisional biopsy unless there is a clear clinical and cytological evidence of malignancy which can not be conclusively categorized on cytological features. As there is 90% chance that a solitary parotid mass is a pleomorphic adenoma Incisional biopsy is contraindicated as a primary investigation to avoid tumor implantation in the surrounding skin.[13]

Frozen section

Frozen section is the process of preparing histologic sections for microscopic examination from frozen diseased tissues. It was first introduced in Holland by de Reimer in 1818. However its use intraoperatively became acceptable after invention of the cryostat during 1940's and 1950's.[11] The overall accuracy of frozen section diagnoses in salivary gland tumors is 96.2% which is slightly low as compared to frozen section diagnoses from other sites of the body which is 98.6%. However, accuracy rate for benign salivary neoplasms is 98.8% and for malignant neoplasms is 85.7%. In a study by Wheelis and Yarington, out of 256 frozen section results they noted a 5%

error in diagnosing benign as malignant and 4 instances of incorrectly diagnosing cancer. The tumors most commonly associated with false negative diagnosis are mucoepidermoid carcinoma (32%), acinic cell carcinoma (18%), adenoid cystic carcinoma (16%) and malignant mixed tumor (16%). Many false negative diagnoses are associated with poor sampling by surgeon or pathologist. Hence, the entire specimen should be submitted to the pathologist so that he can select the area to freeze. Carcinomas arising in pleomorphic adenomas are often localized to one region and may infiltrate focally and hence prone to false negative diagnoses. Similarly, acinic cell carcinoma and mucoepidermoid carcinomas appear cystic and are prone to being diagnosed as benign. Hence it is essential to sample necrotic, solid or cystic portions of the specimen to reduce the incidence of false negative diagnoses. If a tumor, however, is encapsulated completely and grossly uniform in appearance and the frozen section reveals a classical histologic pattern a specific diagnosis can be rendered. However it should be remembered that a therapeutic decision should not be made based on frozen section diagnosis alone and clinical features should also be considered while deciding on the treatment planning.[11]

Histopathological diagnosis of salivary gland tumors is often challenging, especially when it is done with FNAC. Clinicians make fanatic efforts to diagnose these lesions preoperatively. However, what is important is to differentiate malignant and benign tumors preoperatively. Subtyping of malignant tumors does not usually influence treatment plan except in specific entities like Adenoid Cystic carcinoma where perineural spread is common. For rest of the tumors, clinical presentation, behavior and cytological and histopathological evidence of malignancy is sufficient to draw a treatment plan as all these tumors need more aggressive treatment and addressing to the metastatic tumor as well. For example, in case of malignant tumor involving parotid gland with clinical evidence of seventh nerve involvement, total parotidectomy with sacrifice of facial nerve is indicated. However, in case of benign tumors or in malignant tumors where facial nerve is not involved clinically, facial nerve sparing surgery is performed. Lymph node metastasis should be addressed with appropriate neck dissection and role of chemotherapy and/or radiotherapy depends on histopathological typing, clinical behavior and extent and evidence of regional and distant metastasis. Hence to conclude, rather than histopathological diagnosis, preoperatively it is enough to know for the surgeon to know if it is benign or malignant.

References

1. Batsakis JG, Regezi JA. The pathology of head and neck tumors: Salivary glands, Part 1. Head Neck Surg. 1978;1:59.

2. Puterman M, Goldstein J. Primary lymph node Kaposi's sarcoma of the parotid gland. Head Neck Surg. 1983;5:535.
3. Eberle RC. Parotid tumors. George GA (Ed). Current Therapy in Otolaryngology – Head and Neck Surgery. 5th edn. pp.232-8.
4. Norman JE, McGurk M. Salivary Gland Imaging. Morse MH (Ed). Color atlas and text of Salivary glands diseases, disorders and surgery. Mosby – Wolfe, Spain 1995.pp.105-27.
5. Lowman RM, Cheng GK. Diagnostic Roentgenology. Rankow RM, Polayes IM, (Eds). Diseases of Salivary glands. WB Saunders, Philadelphia; 1976;4:54-98.
6. Prof. Col Dr Ranajit Sen. Salivary gland neoplasms. Surgery for Oral and Maxillofacial cysts and tumors. Moumita Sen Publishers, Kolkata. 2002;4: 238-76.
7. DelBalso A. Salivary imaging. Oral and Maxillofacial Surg Clin N Am. 1995; 7(3):387-422.
8. Hanna EY, Suen JY. The Parotid Neoplasm. Controversies in Otolaryngology. Pensak ML. (Ed) Publication Thieme; New York. 2001;22(66):348-54.
9. Taylor & Francis. Acta Oto-Laryngologica. 1998;118(suppl 538): 214-20.
10. Lore JM Jr, Medina JE. The parotid salivary gland and management of malignant salivary gland neoplasia. An atlas of head and neck surgery. 4th edn Elsevier Saunders 2005;7:861-91.
11. Auclair PL, Ellis GL, Douglas GR, Wenig BM, Janney CG. Salivary gland neoplasms: General considerations. Ellis GL (Ed). Surgical pathology of the salivary glands. WB Saunders, Philadelphia. 1991;9:135-64.
12. Batsakis JG. Tumors of the head and neck – Clinical and pathological considerations 2nd edn. Williams and Wilkins, Baltimore. 1979;1.
13. John Watkinson, Mark Gaze, Janet Wilson. Tumors of the major salivary glands. Stell and Maran's Head and Neck Surgery. 4th edn butterworth Heinemann; Oxford. 2000;22:441-58.
14. Robert Marx. Incisional Parotid biopsy for the diagnosis of systemic disease. Oral and Maxillofac Surg Clin of N Am. 1995;7(3):505-6.

Non-neoplastic diseases

chapter 7

Non-neoplastic disorders affecting the salivary glands are mainly inflammatory and noninflammatory. Although both major as well as minor salivary glands are afflicted by these disorders, the major salivary glands are most commonly affected. Proper diagnosis of these diseases needs a thorough understanding and knowledge of various disorders affecting these glands. Acute inflammatory conditions generally can be diagnosed based on history and clinical examination alone whereas chronic inflammatory diseases and granulomatous disorders require supplementation with laboratory tests, imaging and or histopathological examination. Therapy ranges from medicinal to surgical depending on the condition and is many a time only symptomatic and supportive.

Inflammatory disorders affecting the salivary glands may be acute or chronic depending on the course of the disease condition. They may also be suppurative or non-suppurative. They are bacterial, viral or fungal in origin. The bacterial infections may be specific (tuberculosis, actinomycosis) or nonspecific such as suppurative infections.

The bacterial diseases can be secondary to:
1. Ductal anamolies
2. Obstructive ductal conditions like sialolithiasis (calculus) or strictures
3. Hematogenous infections
4. Secondary to dehydration (uremia, liver failure, diabetes, exanthematous fevers)
5. Immunosupressed states
6. Secondary to viral infections like mumps.

The infections result secondary to stasis of salivary flow, which in turn facilitates the retrograde spread of the bacteria from oral cavity to the gland through the duct. Poor oral hygiene is one of the predisposing factors for the suppurative sialoadentis

Acute bacterial sialadenitis

Acute infection can involve any salivary gland, although the major glands are affected more commonly than minor glands. The earliest report of acute bacterial sialadenitis was in 1828, wherein a 71 year old gentleman with a parotid infection progressed to gangrene.[1] However, it was not until 1881, when President Garfield died from acute parotitis following an abdominal surgery and associated dehydration, that awareness regarding this entity was increased.[1] The most commonly affected gland is the parotid.[1] Early in the 20th century, surgeons were hesitant to incise and drain parotid abscesses and frequently used ineffective conservative measures until the process was irreversible. They feared the consequences of the unsightly scar and facial paralysis.

Epidemiology

Acute parotitis usually occurs in debilitated patients who are chronically ill or have undergone a surgical procedure or are convalescing from a prolonged febrile episode. It predominantly occurs in the sixth and seventh decades of life. However, cases are also reported in infancy. Both the sexes are equally affected.[2] Historically, mortality rates were as high as 80% in the 1800's before the advent of antibiotics.[1] However, these days mortality rate has drastically reduced to 20 to 50%.[1-3]

Etiologic factors

Most commonly, parotitis occurs secondary to a debilitating systemic illness. Predisposing factors include:
1. Severe dehydration, usually in postoperative patients.
2. Elderly population is at a higher risk for bacterial parotitis due to decrease in the quantity of salivary secretions.
3. Poor oral hygiene.
4. Reduced host resistance, as in debilitating illnesses such as hepatic failure, renal failure, diabetes mellitus, hypothyroidism, malnutrition, Sjogren's syndrome, depression, anorexia or bulimia, hyperuricemia, hyperlipoproteinemia, cystic fibrosis, lead intoxication, cushing's disease.[1]
5. Immunosuppressed host.
6. HIV associated parotitis.
7. Medications which induce systemic dehydration such as antihypertensives, diuretics, tricyclic antidepressants, pheno-thiazines, betablockers, barbiturates, anticholinergics.[1]
8. Radiotherapy for head and neck cancer.
9. Mechanical obstruction to salivary flow

Pathogenesis

Mode of spread of organisms into the salivary glands may be caused by a combination of factors that enhance ascension of oral bacteria through the salivary ducts viz stenson's and wharton's ducts.[4,5] It mainly occurs by two important physiologic mechanisms.[1] First one is retrograde contamination of salivary ducts and parenchymal tissues by oral microflora which provides a bacterial source of infection. Second one is stasis of salivary flow through the ducts and parenchyma which promotes acute suppurative infection. This process can affect any major gland but, parotid gland is most commonly affected.[1]

Predilection of parotid gland is due to various physiologic and anatomic factors. Parotid saliva is primarily serous whereas submandibular and sublingual glands secrete mucous saliva. Mucous saliva has lysosomes, IgA antibodies which have antimicrobial activity. Also, it contains sialic acid which agglutinates bacteria and reduces their adherence to host tissue. Specific glycoproteins in mucins bind epithelial cells and hence inhibit bacterial attachment selectively.[6]

Sialolithiasis produces mechanical obstruction of the duct with salivary stasis leading to subsequent salivary gland inflammation. However, in spite of higher frequency of sialolithiasis in sub-mandibular duct and gland, parotid gland is affected most commonly.

Bacteriology

Staphylococcus aureus is the most common causative organism for acute suppurative parotitis, being cultured in 50 to 80% of the cases. Streptococcal species including *Streptococcus pneumoniae* and *Streptococcus pyogenes* (β hemolytic streptococci) as well as Hemophilus influenza are also commonly involved in causation of acute bacterial sialadenitis.[7] According to RAAD et al, the presence of fibronectin in saliva promotes adherence of *Staphylococcus* and *Streptococcus* species.[3]

In addition to these routinely cultured organisms, suppurative sialadenitis has also been reported in the submandibular gland due to infection by Methicillin resistant *Staphylococcus aureus* (MRSA) in a premature neonate.[8] Anaerobic bacteria have also been implicated as causative organisms in two cases of suppurative sialadenitis in newborns and two by Brook et al.[9]

Other organisms which might result into the suppurative sialadenitis include peptostreptococcus species, Prevotella species, Porphyromonas species, Fusobacterium nucleatum, *Mycobacterium tuberculosis*, *Mycobacterium avium-intracellulare*. Rarely, Pseudomonas aeruginosa, *E. coli*, Proteus species, Salmonella species, Klebsiella species, Actinobacillus species and Actinomyces species may also result into suppurative sialadenitis.[10]

Clinical features

Systemic sepsis is more commonly associated with parotid gland infections as compared to submandibular gland infections. This is suggestive of an increased propensity of parotitis to occur in debilitated patients. Signs and symptoms of acute suppurative sialadenitis are as follows:

Non-neoplastic diseases 57

1. Localized symptoms such as sudden onset of pain and swelling over affected gland. Usually it is unilateral, but in 10 to 25% cases it may be bilateral.[3] **(Figure 7.2)**.
2. Pain is exacerbated by meals or sight and smell of food i.e. increase in severity with gustation.
3. General constitutional signs and symptoms like high grade fever, malaise, and body ache, leucocytosis are seen. The signs of dehydration may be present. Patients appear toxic and may also have deliriums **(Figures 7.1A and B)**.
4. The local signs are diffuse inflammatory swelling, induration, erythema, edema and extreme tenderness over the parotid area in cases of parotid sialadenitis and over the submandibular triangle in case submandibular gland is affected **(Figure 7.1C)**. The skin becomes tense, glossy and erythematous. The ear lobule gets lifted, which is the pathognomonic sign of parotid swelling **(Figure 7.1D)**. However, it is not seen in the very early stages of the disease.

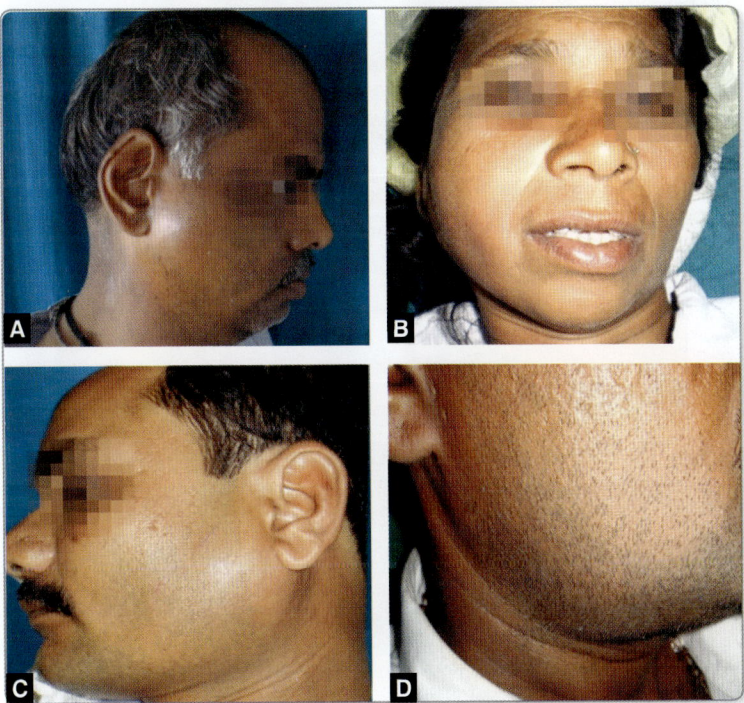

Figures 7.1A to D Unilateral acute bacterial parotitis; (A) Tense and shiny swelling in preauricular area; (B) Toxic appearance of patient with minimal swelling over right angle region; (C) Lifting of ear lobule suggestive of parotid gland swelling (sialadenitis); (D) Submandibular sialadenitis with swelling in submandibular triangle

58 Salivary gland pathologies

5. The ducts as well as salivary caruncle situated on the buccal mucosa opposite the maxillary second molar (opening of Stenson's duct) and in the floor of the mouth lateral to the lingual frenulum (opening of the Wharton's duct) is inflamed and edematous **(Figure 7.2)**.
6. The salivary flow is diminished which can be appreciated on milking the gland. Oral cavity also appears dry, crusted and skin turgor may be lost.
7. Milking of the gland may lead to purulent discharge from the orifice in case the abscess is already formed **(Figure 7.3)**. Early cases do not yield pus on milking of gland.

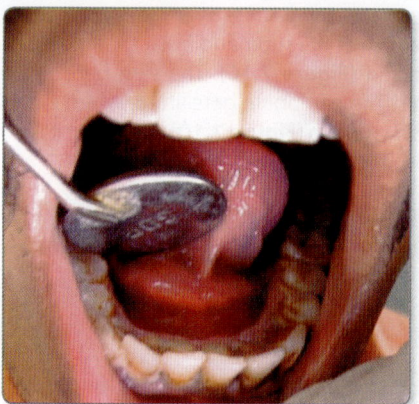

Figure 7.2 Inflammation of Wharton's duct

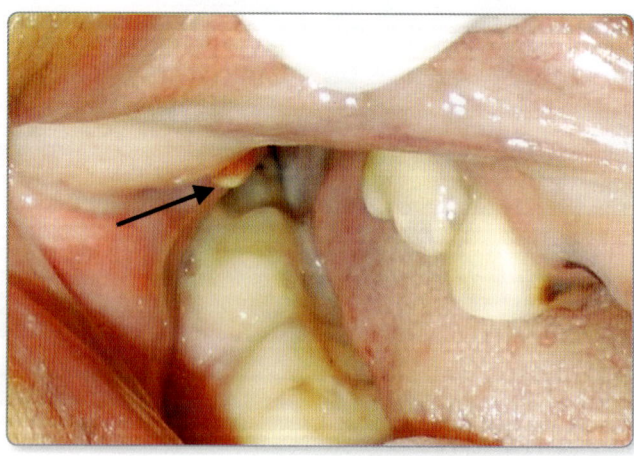

Figure 7.3 Pus expressed at the salivary caruncle

8. A salivary calculus might also be palpable along the course of the duct.
9. Due to the presence of the dense fascia around the parotid gland (Parotideomassetric fascia), the swellings are not fluctuant and are extremely painful due to the mounting pressure as the fascia is non yeilding. This mounting pressure leads to ischemic necrosis of the gland and the abscess may spontaneously burst in the external auditory canal.
10. The Stenson's duct when palpated over the clenched masseter muscle feels cord like due to sialadenosis, i.e. inflammation of the duct.

Investigations

Diagnosis of acute suppurative sialadenitis is mainly clinical. Laboratory investigations and diagnostic imaging rarely plays any role. They are indicated if the patient fails to respond to conventional therapy. However, a screening radiograph (OPG) should be obtained to rule out any sialolith which could have resulted in the infection.

After thorough clinical examination, routine laboratory evaluation of the patient is done. Blood investigations are suggestive of leukocytosis with neutrophilia. Serum amylase is within normal limits. Imaging studies are not an absolute emergency but should be performed to rule out any obstructive pathology such as calculus. Plain X-rays can be done. To rule out a deep seated abscess formation, USG, CT scan or MRI scan can be performed. Sialography is contraindicated in cases of acute suppurative sialadenitis as it may aggrevate the infection and leads to the necrosis of the gland. Aspiration from the swollen inflamed gland rarely yields pus. The culture and sensitivity studies of the pus specimen from the duct by taking a swab after milking the gland may help in planning the antibiotic therapy.

Management

Treatment is directed towards reversal of underlying medical condition responsible for the infection as well as controlling the active infection and preventing it from progressing. Hence the treatment is aimed at symptomatic relief as well as definitive management of the underlying cause and comprises of medicinal, supportive and surgical line of management.

Medicinal management comprises of stoppage of anti-sialogogue medication if any and administration of empirical antimicrobial therapy directed towards gram positive and anaerobic organisms. Most of the cultured organisms produce beta-lactamase or penicillinase.[3] Hence, beta-lactamase inhibitor containing antimicrobial therapy of choice include augmented penicillins containing clavulinic acid or sulbactam. Also, antistaphylococcal penicillins (oxacillin, dicloxacillin, methicillin) and second generation cephalosporins which are penicillinase resistant may be used. Addition of metronidazole is also advocated.[11] Depending on whether

60 Salivary gland pathologies

case is treated on OPD or IPD basis, oral or parentral drugs are administered respectively.

Supportive care includes hydration of patient either orally or parentrally. Use of antiseptic mouth wash for maintenance of oral hygiene and reducing oral bacterial count is advocated. Warm saline rinses and compresses can be used. Sialogogues, i.e. sour candies are use along with gentle massage to drain the gland.[12] The infection usually resolves with this treatment. Under no circumstances should the duct be probed or sialography performed to avoid the infection from being forced proximally deep into the parenchymal tissue.[13]

However, one should not wait for a long-time if treatment response is slow for the localizing signs of the infection such as fluctuation to occur. Instead a prompt incision and drainage/ decompression should be undertaken if medicinal management does not result in improvement within two days. This relieves internal pressure and not only provides symptomatic relief from pain but also helps to prevent ischemic necrosis of the gland. The best way of draining the parotid abscess is by placing an incision parallel to the branches of the facial nerve to avoid injury to them. The preauricular incision and blunt dissection with multiple incisions into the parotid fascia parallel to the facial nerve branches, to drain the abscess gives good cosmetic results. However, a retromandibilar incision can also be given and dissection carried into the parotideomasseteric fascia to drain the pus **(Figure 7.4)**. This incision also gives an adequate access to incise the parotid fascia and also avoids trauma to facial nerve branches when dissection is carried out over the masseter muscle. In addition, it also provides a gravity dependent drainage. A drain can be maintained to keep the drainage site patent.

Other most important aspect of management of this condition is to diagnose the etiologic factor responsible and manage it. If a salivary calculus

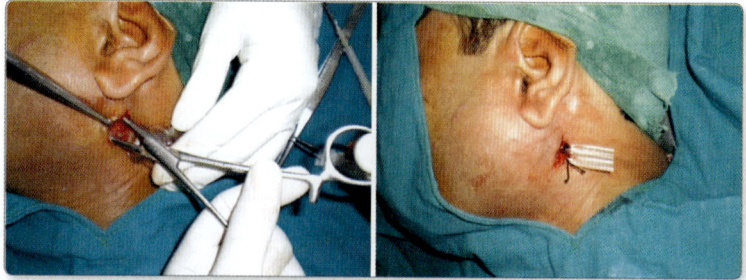

Figure 7.4 Incision and drainage of parotid abscess by retromandibular incision

is found on imaging studies, it should be removed as soon as possible failing which the infection might not subside or may enter into a chronic phase.

Complications

Complications might result due to local spread of infection to adjacent tissue spaces or due to its spread through the hematogenous route. If acute bacterial parotitis is not drained early during the course of its progression, the mounting pressure due to unyielding nature of the fascial covering leads to an increased parenchymal damage, which undergoes necrosis and abscess formation. **Figure 7.5** show a similar case wherein the local practitioner waited 10 days for the symptoms to subside with medical management before referring the patient.

Still, if there is a delay in draining the abscess, it might rupture into the external auditory canal, temporomandibular joint or may spread into the adjacent parapharyngeal spaces through the weak area of the fascia on the deep aspect.[3,14] It may also result into osteomyelitis of the TMJ and mandible and thrombophlebitis of the retromandibular or facial vein.[3,14]

If the abscess bursts into the parapharyngeal spaces may result into airway obstruction, spread along the anterior Lincoln's highway into the anterior mediastinum, internal jugular vein thrombosis, carotid artery erosion. Pneumonia might result if the abscess bursts into the airway. Guardia et al have reported a fatal necrotizing mediastinitis secondary to acute suppurative parotitis.[15] Rarely a reversible facial nerve weakness results due to perineuritis or direct neural compression which resolves after the parotitis is treated adequately.[16,17]

Due to systemic compromise of most of the patients, it can lead to sepsis which can progress to septic shock or multi organ failure which is usually fatal.[1]

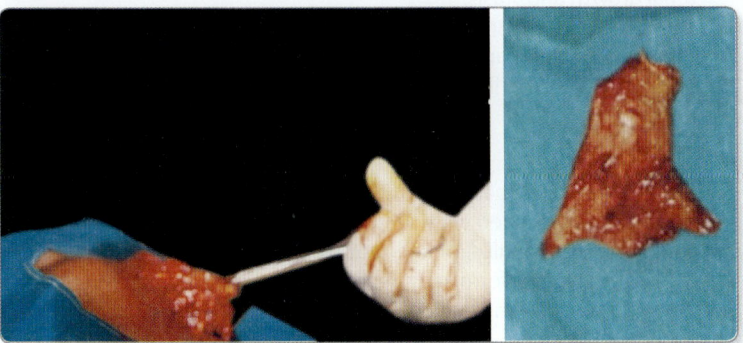

Figure 7.5 Necrosed parotid gland due to delay of 10 days in establishing drainage (*Courtesy:* Dr Suhas Jajoo)

Chronic bacterial sialadenitis

It is also known as chronic recurrent sialadenitis. It is characterized by unilateral or bilateral swellings with periodic episodic relapsing and remitting swellings of the major salivary glands.[12] Like acute sialadenitis, chronic sialadenitis is also more common in the parotid gland than other salivary glands.[18]

Etiology

The etiology of chronic sialadenitis is multifactorial. Salivary stasis is the most common preceding event which predisposes the gland to infection. Acute suppurative sialadenitis causes permanent damage to gland parenchyma which results into chronic sialadenitis.[18] Inflammation of the gland causes multifocal wall irregularities which cause stricture formation.[19] Multiple strictures also results into chronic sialadenitis due to salivary stasis.[12]

Clinical features

1. There is a sudden onset of diffuse parotid swelling, typically unilateral but occasionally bilateral, with varying degrees of discomfort. There is no association with meals or seasons suggesting no obstructive or allergic phenomenon.[20] However, previous concept of rice DH was that a patient with chronic sialadenitis had a history of recurrent painful gland enlargement and that it aggravated on eating.[18]
2. Swelling may persist for days, weeks or months and is associated with low-grade fever.
3. Quiescent period between attacks can vary from months to years.
4. Pus is absent but a type of material referred to as 'mucopus' is produced which blocks the duct and causes salivary stasis and favors further bacterial growth and stasis.
5. Salivary gland milking may demonstrate scanty saliva. Up to 80% of these patients end up with xerostomia.
6. Two forms are described in literature, viz adult and juvenile forms.

Microbiology

The adult form is associated with *Staphylococcus aureus* infection and juvenile form is associated with *Streptococcus viridians*. In the juvenile form, children particularly males, of age group 3 to 6 years are more commonly affected. The juvenile form may recover spontaneously at puberty with functional recovery of the gland.

Diagnosis

As with acute phase, a detailed history and a thorough clinical evaluation of the patient are of immense value in establishing a diagnosis. A screening radiograph is taken to rule out any sialoloith. Sialography using a water soluble dye is of use in studying the ductal pattern. It starts as punctuate sialectasis with dilatation of peripheral ducts and later progresses to sausage like dilatation of the duct due to dilatations and strictures.[19] MRI is more specific than CT; however, sialo-MRI is more specific and accurate.[12]

Management

There are two important elements of therapy. The first one is to reduce or eliminate the inflammation of the gland by using short term corticosteroids. Unless there is an acute exacerbation, antibiotics play no role.[12] The second goal of therapy is to clear the precipitated serum proteins within the intraductal system.[12] This is performed by increasing the salivary flow by use of sialogogues and warm compresses.[19] The most effective technique to achieve an increased salivary flow is use of sialoendoscope. Even patients with atleast one acute episode per year should also be considered for sialoendoscopy.[19] The sialoendoscope is advanced in the duct until it meets obstruction. Advancement of scope is done with continuous normal saline lavage which helps in visualization of ductal system and in dilating the strictures within the duct. The sialoballon may be used to dilate the strictures of the duct. A stent may be inserted to assist in preventing redevelopment of strictures over a four week period.[19] The other recommended treatments include periodic ductal dilatation, ligation of duct, total gland irradiation, tympanic neurectomy and excision of the gland.[18] Superficial parotidectomy with facial nerve preservation can also be considered in case of chronic pain, provided imaging studies determine the involvement of superficial lobe.[12]

Complications

Chronic recurrent parotitis may eventually lead to development of benign lymphoepithelial lesion.[21] These can further progress to lymphoproliferative disorders like Non-Hodgkins lymphoma, carcinoma or pseudolymphoma.

Obstructive disorders of the salivary glands

Obstructive disorders of salivary glands result from sialolithiasis, strictures and mucoceles and salivary cysts.[22]

Sialolithiasis

Sialolithiasis is the most common cause of obstruction in major salivary glands[23] and one of the most common pathologies associated with salivary glands and is the major cause for salivary gland dysfunction.[24] This is a chronic and recurring disease seen most commonly in the middle and later decades of life.[22,24] Not all cases become symptomatic. Only those cases with superadded infection and inflammation of the gland and duct result into pain.

Epidemiology

Sialolithiasis accounts for 50% of major salivary gland disease.[22] However, the prevalence of symptomatic salivary calculi may be 0.45%. There is a slight male preponderance, and the peak incidence is between the ages of 30 and 60.[22,25] However, it can be seen in all age groups right from infants to elderly.[24] The commonest site is the submandibular gland where 80 to 90% of calculi are found, 5 to 10% are found in the parotid gland and approximately 5% in the sublingual and other minor salivary glands.[22,23] The ratio of occurrence of submandibular to parotid sialolith is from as low as 4:1 to 12:1.[24]

Etiologic factors

The exact cause of sialolithiasis is unknown. However, certain conditions and anatomic peculiarities predispose the glands to this condition. Predisposition to calculus formation is salivary stasis in the gland or duct. In case of parotid gland the most common site is the right angle bend of the Stenson's duct where it pierces the buccinator muscle at the anterior border of the masseter. Similarly, the submandibular duct has a 90^0 bend at the posterior border of the mylohyoid muscle which is the most common site for calculus formation.

Chronic sialadenitis is known to cause intraductal and intraglandular concretions which promotes calculus formation.[24]

Partial obstruction of gland also increases the propensity to calculus formation. However, completely obstructed gland does not show calculus formation due to depletion of calcium secretory granules in the acini and low lithogenic potential of the saliva.[26]

The primary etiologic factors include:[2]
1. Neurohumoral condition leading to salivary stagnation
2. Nidus or matrix for stone formation
3. Metabolic mechanism favoring precipitation of salivary salts into the matrix in presence of coexisting inflammation.

Stone formation is not associated with any systemic abnormalities of calcium metabolism. Gout is the only systemic illness known to predispose to salivary stone formation.[27] Lustmann et al have found a correlation between sialolithiasis and nephrolithiasis in 10% of the patients.[28] Berini L et al have found a lower correlation of 4% cases.[29]

Pathophysiology

Intermittent stasis of salivary secretion is necessary for stone formation. This stasis results into change in the mucoid element of saliva which forms a gel. This gel forms a framework for deposition of salts and organic substances creating a stone. Unknown metabolic phenomenon causes increase in the salivary bicarbonate content which alters the calcium phosphate solubility and leads to precipitation of calcium and phosphate ions.[24] The composition of salivary calculi is predominantly calcium phosphate and carbonate in the form of hydroxyapatite with small quantity of magnesium, potassium and ammonium. Majority of stones are formed from phosphate and oxalate salts with a clear distinction between submandibular and parotid stones both in frequency and composition. Parotid gland stones contain more acidic mineral phases, such as brushite and octacalcium phosphate and contain about 70% more organic matrix, 40% more protein and 54% more lipids. The organic matrix of submandibular stones, however, is richer in protein and has a higher (13%) content of lipids. They grow by deposition and range in size from 0.1 mm to 30 mm.[22] Salivary calculi may mature in the salivary duct system extraglandularly or intraglandularly. Multiple calculi may be present in one gland or bilateral sialoliths may occur.[2]

The submandibular glandular system is more susceptible to sialolith formation than parotid due to its unique physiologic and anatomic peculiarities. Physiologically the saliva secreted by the submandibular gland is more alkaline. Also, it contains a greater concentration of calcium and phosphate salts, mainly apatites. The relative alkalinity along with alteration in salivary calcium– phosphorous ratio causes the salivary apatite to exceed its solubility product and precipitation occurs.[2] In addition, mucus content of the submandibular gland is under control of autonomic nervous system and its secretions are more viscous than parotid secretions. So also, the Wharton's duct is longer than the Stenson's duct and the submandibular gland is situated at a lower level than the opening of the duct. Hence, the duct has to follow an uphill, tortuous course and drain against gravity. So, stagnation of secretions is more common than parotid gland.

Other major difference between submandibular and parotid calculi is that in case of submandibular gland, the calculus forms primarily and occurrence of sialadenitis is secondary to the resultant stagnation of salivary secretions due to retrograde infection. In case of parotid gland, primary pathology is glandular or ductal inflammation which predisposes to calculus formation.[2] In the parotid gland stones are most commonly located at the hilum or parenchyma whereas submandibular sialoliths develop in the duct.[28]

The calculi are laminated in morphology with laminations being irregular suggestive of intermittent deposition of salts.

Clinical features

Patients present with swelling **(Figure 7.6A)** in most of the cases which is usually associated with pain in most of the cases but might even be painless. However, in a few cases pain is the only presenting symptom. Ellies et al found 59% cases with a painful swelling, 29% cases with painless swelling and 12% cases with only pain.[30]

The patient typically has a recurrent salivary colic and spasmodic pains upon eating. The patient may have repeated infections as well as abscess formations.[24] Symptoms of patient depend on relative obstruction to salivary flow.[24] The duct and orifice may be inflamed due to the prevailing infection **(Figure 7.6B)**. Sometimes typically the sialolith is expelled out of the gland through the duct and is seen at the duct orifice **(Figures 7.7A and B)**.

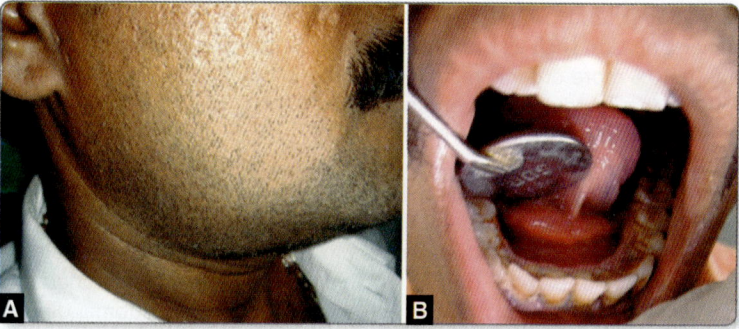

Figures 7.6A and B (A) Extraoral swelling associated with sialolith of Wharton's duct; (B) Inflammation of Wharton's duct

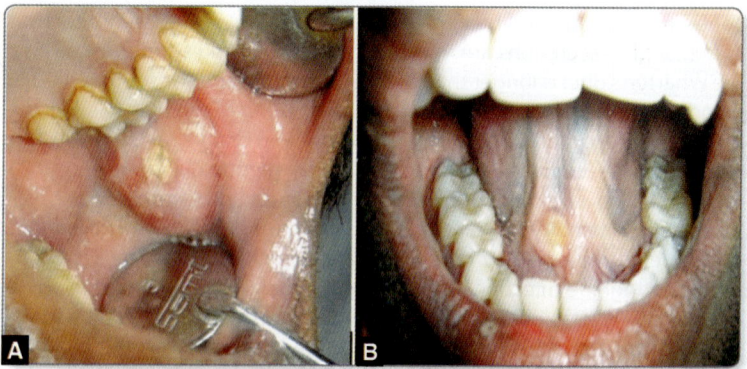

Figures 7.7A and B (A) Sialolith present at the parotid papilla on the cheek; (B) Sialolith present at the sublingual caruncle in the floor of mouth

Diagnosis

Like all disorders, a detailed history and thorough clinical examination are mandatory to diagnosis of sialolithiasis. Bimanual palpation of the glands should be done.

A screening radiograph (OPG) should be taken which can be followed by definitive plain radiographs, ultrasonography, CT scan, MRI. A occlusal radiograph is used in submandibular sialolithiasis and a PA puffed cheek view is used in diagnosis of Parotid calculus. The plain radiographs will detect presence of radiopaque calculi **(Figures 7.8A to E)**. The so called 'comma' area is not properly visualized by means of an occlusal film because the accurate positioning of the film causes the patient to gag.[2] However, the parotid stones are more commonly radiolucent and are missed on plain radiographs. Also, presence of phleboliths, arterial atherosclerosis of lingual artery or calcified cervical lymph node mimic sialoliths.[24,26]

Sialography is said to be the mainstay for diagnosis of sialoliths. It can be used with plain radiographs or digital subtraction sialography can be done. It has a sensitivity of 95 to 100% and detects radiolucent stones also.[24] Sialograms are said to be 100% effective in detecting ductal and intraglandular calculi.[31] However, sialography is contraindicated in case of acute infection and in case the sialolith is already diagnosed on a plain radiograph and is situated in the oral part of the Wharton's duct. Also, if a lipophilic dye is used, there are chances of pushing the calculus much deeper if more pressure is applied while injecting the dye. The added advantage

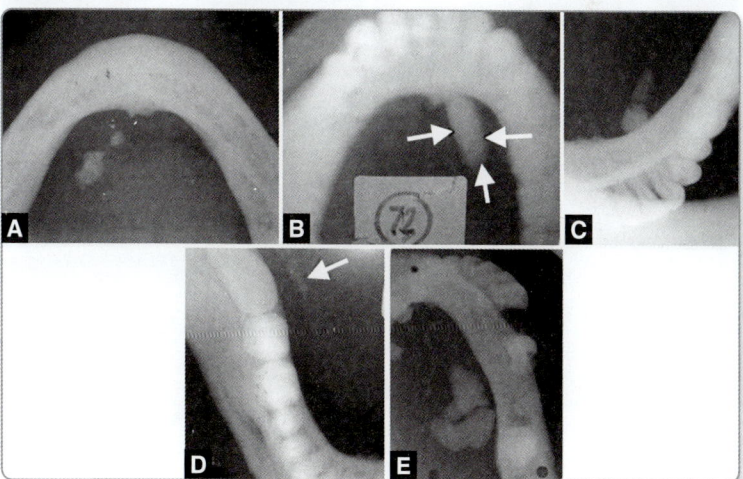

Figures 7.8A to E Occlusal radiograhs showing radiopaque calculus (A to D) in Wharton's duct and (E) in the submandibular gland

68 Salivary gland pathologies

of sialogram is that, in addition to detecting obstructive pathology, it also gives information regarding condition of gland.

Management

In case of small stones, conservative treatment can be tried. The patient should be well hydrated. Local heat application, gland massage and sialogoques may assist in flushing out the stone. In case of an evident swelling associated with a sialolith, infection of the gland must be assumed and antibiotic therapy should be started.[24] Stones less than 2 mm in size can be expected to be expelled from the duct by conservative means with only dilatation of the punctum.

The surgical management depends on the anatomic location of the calculus. If the calculus is within one centimeter of the punctum, filleting of the duct can be done. Under local anesthesia, the ostium and duct is dilated with a lacrimal probe and the duct is cut with an iris scissor with one blade within the duct and the other on the mucosa of the floor of the mouth. After opening the duct, the stone can be grasped with forceps and extracted. The gland is milked to remove any debris within the duct. The wound is left unsutured.[24]

Submandibular calculi which are slightly deeper but easily palpable in the duct and within two centimeters from the duct orifice can be approached transorally **(Figure 7.9)**. A silk suture is placed proximal to the

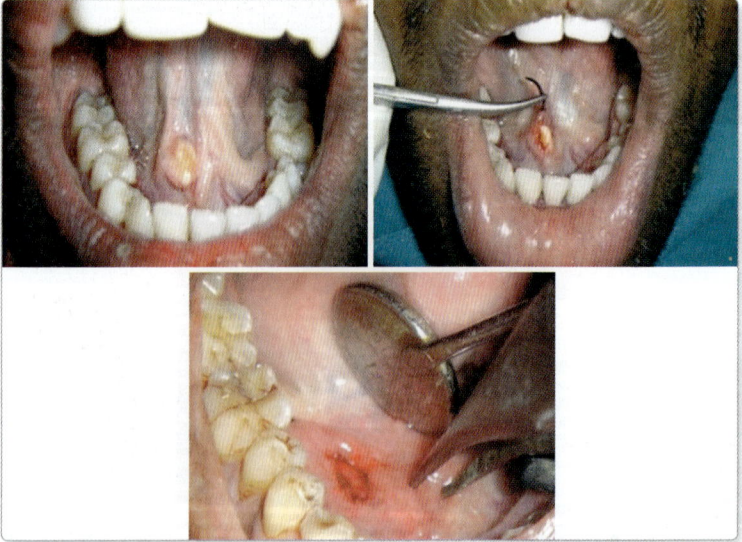

Figure 7.9 Transoral surgical management of submandibular calculus

calculus to avoid slipping of the calculus deeper into the duct. An incision is placed directly over the calculus and the calculus retrieved. The duct is not sutured to avoid stricture formation. Care should be taken to avoid damage to the lingual nerve which is in close proximity to the duct posteriorly.

Submandibular calculus which is present in a deeper location warrants a sialadenectomy which can be performed through transoral or transcervical approach.[26]

Parotid stone removal is more problematic.[24] In case of parotid stones, only those calculi which are situated distal to the masseter muscle can be removed transorally. Rest of the calculi requires a parotidectomy. Thus, only around 1.5 cm of the duct is amenable to intraoral surgery. The duct lateral to the masseter cannot be approached transorally.[24] Parotid gland is more prone to stricture formation, after removal of the calculus.[26] An extraoral approach involving an incision directly onto the calculus has been described by Baurmash et al. The calculus which is larger than 1.5 cm and located between the hilum of the gland and the anterior bend of the duct lateral to the masseter muscle can be managed by this approach. An intraductal probe is placed in the stenson's duct. The stenson's duct is marked from the earlobe to the point where the intraductal probe can be felt. A 2 cm incision is placed on this line and the duct is identified using blunt dissection. Care should be taken to avoid damage to the buccal branch of the facial nerve which is close approximation to the duct. The duct is reconstructed after removal of the stone and wound is closed. With this approach, a parotidectomy can be avoided.[32] However; parotidectomy is the mainstay of surgical management of parotid sialoliths which are intraglandular and hilar in location.[24]

Newer alternative modalities of management include extracorporeal shock wave lithotripsy and use of sialoendoscopy. Lithotripsy reduces calculi to small fragments that are then flushed out of the duct with spontaneous salivation or use of secretogogue.[26] Extracorporeal lithotripsy (ECL) was introduced in the early 1980s for management of urinary stones. In 1989, it was first successfully used in the management of parotid sialolith.[33]

There are three types of lithotripters used for urinary lithiasis viz hydroelectric, electromagnetic, piezoelectric. The first two are unable to focus into small anatomic areas, as well as cause collateral injury to adjacent tissue. The piezoelectric lithotripter, introduced in 1986, produces a narrow spot size and lends itself to salivary stone management. However, the primary requirement for salivary stone lithotripsy is a functional gland which produces saliva which will clear the fragmented stone. A 'gum test' which involves chewing of a sour gum can be done to test the functionality of the salivary gland. If the salivary secretions are normal, a visible swelling in the region of the gland will be noticed. If the test is negative, the patient cannot be taken up for lithotripsy. ECL can be performed without local or general anesthesia. ECL appears to be the most effective treatment for parotid sialolith.[24] Iro et al have found that 50% patients were rendered free of calculi, 26% free of symptoms but had small fragments of calculi in the ductal system.[34] ECL can fragment stones of any composition.[24] Ottaviani et al have recommended lithotripsy for patients with parotid stones in whom conservative treatment has failed, before planning any surgical intervention.[35] In case of submandibular stones, if the sialolith is amenable to intraoral surgical removal, it is by far the best option. An intraglandular sialolith below 7 mm may be amenable to lithotripsy. However, a relatively lower stone free rate is seen after submandibular gland lithotripsy.[35]

Viral infections of salivary glands

Viral infections of the salivary glands occur through hematogenous dissemination of infection. However, a retrogrde ductal migration of infection also occurs. These infections are not always locally symptomatic.[26] Viral infections include mumps and HIV parotitis.

Mumps

It is also known as "epidemic parotitis". Mumps classically defines an acute nonsuppurative viral parotitis caused by paramyxovirus. However, a broad range of viruses have been identified as etiologic factors.[1,26] The term "Mumps" is derived from the Danish word "Mompen" which means mumbling (like an old man) and describes the difficulty with speech because of inflammation and trismus.[1]

Pathogenesis

They are systemic in onset. The virus is endemic in community and is spread by air-borne droplets which enter the body through the upper respiratory tract. The incubation period is 2 to 3 weeks during which the virus multiplies in the upper respiratory tract or parotid gland. This phase is followed by a 3 to 5 day period of viremia. The virus then localizes to biologically active tissue, such as salivary glands, germinal tissues and CNS.[36] The infection may also affect the submandibular glands, although it has a strong predilection for the parotid gland.[36]

Epidemiology

Mumps is the most common cause of nonsuppurative acute sialadenitis and occurs worldwide.[26] It is highly contagious.[1] The peak incidence of mumps is in the 4 to 6 year old group of children.[37] Eighty five percent of the infections occur in children under the age of 15 years.[36] Adults are rarely infected due to the immunity because of childhood exposure or due to the MMR vaccine.[1]

Non-neoplastic diseases 71

Virology

Classic mumps is acused by a paramyxovirus, an RNA virus related to the influenza and parainfluenza viruses. Other viruses involved in the pathogenesis of mumps include influenza and parainfluenza (types 1 and 3) viruses, coxsackie virus A and B, ECHO virus, lymphocytic choriomeningitic virus.[1]

Clinical features[1]

1. At least around one third of the patients present with prodromal symptoms prior to development of parotitis which include headache, myalgias, arthralgias, anorexia and malaise.
2. The onset of salivary gland involvement starts with an earache, followed by pain localized to the gland, trismus and dysphagia.
3. Pain is exacerbated by salivary stimulation during meals by the sight and smell of food and during chewing.
4. The parotid papilla may be inflamed and puffy.[39]
5. Palpation of the gland reveals a swelling of the gland which may be tense, rubbery[39] and firm with nonpitting type edema.[1,26]
6. The overlying skin is tensed with glazed appearance but erythema or increased temperature may be absent.[1,26]
7. Swelling lasts for 1 to 5 days and can displace the pinna.
8. 75% cases result in bilateral involvement of parotid gland. However, it begins as a unilateral swelling and involves the contra lateral gland after a period of 1 to 5 days.[36]
9. The patient has low grade fever, especially during the prodromal stage.

Diagnosis

It is mainly clinical diagnosis which may be supplemented by laboratory tests. Contrary to acute bacterial parotitis, Mumps typically shows a leukocytopenia with relative lymphocytosis. Serum amylase levels are also raised.[3] It peaks during the first week and start declining in the second or third week and come back to normal during this phase.

Serological studies are necessary to confirm the diagnosis. 'S' or soluble antibodies directed against the nucleoprotein core of the virus, appear within the first week of infection and peak within 2 weeks. 'S' antibodies disappear within 8 to 9 months and are associated with active infection or recent immunization. 'V' or viral antibodies directed against the outer surface hemagglutinin, appear several weeks after the 'S' antibodies and persist at low levels for approximately 5 years following exposure. They are associated with past infection, prior vaccination and late stages of active infection.[1]

If initial serology is noncontributory, a nonparamyxovirus infection may be suspected. Antibody titers against other viruses mentioned before should be obtained. A fourfold rise in antibody titer is diagnostic of active infection. Rarely, the virus can be cultured from blood, saliva, breast milk or cerebrospinal fluid (CSF).[1]

Mumps skin test is not useful in the diagnosis of acute infection because dermal hypersensitivity does not develop until 3 or 4 weeks following viral exposure.[1]

Treatment

As the disease is self-limiting, treatment is primarily supportive, including rest and adequate hydration. Antipyretics and anti-inflammatory medications are beneficial. Live attenuated Jeryl Lynn vaccine is available since 1967, which revolutionized the treatment of mumps. The vaccine is combined with measles and rubella vaccines and is administered as a single vaccine in a single subcutaneous dose after 12 months of age. Measurable antibody titre is present in 90% cases.[1] Infections are also reported in immunized patients and are probably salivary infection with a nonparamyxovirus or rarely failed vaccination.[38] The vaccine is contraindicated in pregnancy, immunocompromised states and allergy to neomycin.[26] unfortunately, the vaccine is not protective to individuals who are already exposed to the virus and are in the incubation stage of the disease.[39]

There are four other vaccines available. However, they are either effective or have a lower safety profile when compared with the Jeryl Lynn vaccine. The other vaccines are Urabe, the Rubini, the Leningrad-Zagreb and the Leningrad-3 strains.[40]

Complications

They are not true complications but, are related to systemic nature of the disease. Orchitis is the most common condition complicating paramyxovirus parotitis and occurs in 20 to 30% of males.[36] Oophoritis occurs in only 5% females.[36] Involvement of germinal tissues does not appear to result into sterility as the orchitis is usually unilateral.[1,39] However, sometimes complete sterility may occur.[39] Mastitis affects 30% of females over age 15 years, and has been associated with decreased lactation.[1] This is a rare complication as only 15% cases occur after an age of 15 years. Aseptic meningitis occurs in 10% cases and asymptomatic meningeal inflammation is more common.[36] Five % patients are affected by acute pancreatitis, wherein serum lipase levels are also increased.

Sensorineural hearing loss complicates approximately 0.05 to 4% of patients.[1,36] The onset of deafness is rapid and develops towards the end of parotitis. Tinnitus, aural fullness and vertigo are associated symptoms but they resolve over a period of few weeks. However, the hearing loss is usually permanent and profound.[1] In 80% cases, hearing loss is unilateral. There is no treatment for mumps associated deafness, but cochlear implantation has been tried.[1]

Additional complications include myocarditis, polyarthritis, hemolytic anemia, plasmacytosis, lymphocytic leukemoid reactions and thrombocytopenia.[1] These conditions are self limiting or resolve with or without steroid therapy.

HIV parotitis

HIV is associated with several pathologic processes involving the salivary glands. The most common salivary gland presentation in HIV infected individuals is salivary gland swelling which can be attributed to acute sialadenitis or HIV-associated salivary gland disease (HIV-SGD).[26,41] HIV-SGD is the term used to describe the diffuse enlargement of the salivary glands and affects patients throughout all stages of the disease.[26] In fact, HIV-SGD may be the first presenting sign of HIV.[44] Like most of the salivary diseases, parotid gland is the most frequently affected.

Other pathologic processes associated with HIV include Kaposi's sarcoma and lymphoma and lymphoproliferative and cystic enlargement of major salivary glands with accompanying salivary dysfunction.[26]

Clinically, HIV infected individuals show reduced salivary flow rates. So also, these patients have salivary secretions which contain an increased sodium chloride, lysozyme, peroxidase, lactoferrin, immunoglobulin A levels.[42] However, salivary secretions have shown low concentrations of the virus.[26] HIV-SGD is seen in both adults as well as children inflicted with the disease, being more common in the later.[42]

Parotid gland enlargement is reported to occur in 1 to 10% of the HIV-infected population.[43] It is usually secondary to development of benign lymphoepithelial cysts within the parotid gland.[41]

Clinical features

1. The patients report with a history of gradual, nontender enlargement of one or more salivary glands.
2. The glandular swellings might fluctuate but are usually stable and long standing.
3. Decreased salivary gland function results into xerostomia and sicca symptoms. This sicca symptom complex clinically mimics Sjogren's syndrome and is classified as "Diffuse infiltrative lymphocytosis syndrome (DILS)".[26] DILS is also termed as benign lymphoepithelial cysts (BLEC).
4. DILS is characterized by presence of persistent circulating CD8 lymphocytosis and visceral CD8 lymphocytic infiltration predominantly in the salivary glands and lungs.
5. DILS can be differentiated from Sjogren's syndrome by the evidence of extraglandular involvement of lungs, gastrointestinal tract and kidneys. Also, autoantibodies will be present in case of Sjogren's syndrome.

Evaluation

CT and MRI are used as diagnostic modalities. On CT, the parotid gland shows multiple thin-walled cystic lesions with low attenuation and diffuse lymphadenopathy. The MRI shows homogenous masses of intermediate signal density on proton density and T-2 weighted images.[44]

Management

The medical management involves management of the etiologic condition with antiretroviral therapy such as Zidovudine, maintenance of oral hygiene and use of sialogogues.[26] In patients with DILS and progressive visceral lymphocytic infiltration, corticosteroids and immunosuppressive therapy may be started.[26]

Sclerotherapy with doxycycline has also been used in management of BLEC with definite promise. Although, the treatment modality causes mild edema and/or tenderness, major complications do not result.

Non-infectious inflammatory diseases

The noninfectious inflammatory diseases afflicting the salivary gland include:
1. Mikulicz's disease.
2. Sjögren's syndrome.

Mikulicz's disease

This is also referred to as "Benign lymphoepithelial lesion of Godwin". It is one of the rather uncommon diseases affecting the salivary glands. It was first reported by Johann von Mikulicz in 1892 as a case of chronic symmetrical enlargement of salivary and lacrimal glands.[2] In 1925, Gougerot, a French dermatologist described a condition manifesting with swelling of the salivary and lacrimal glands and associated with dryness of the eyes and mouth. The lesion showed histologic infiltration of lymphocytes. There was also dryness of nose, larynx and occasional decreased thyroid function.[2] In 1927, Mulock Houwer correlated dryness of eyes with rheumatoid arthritis. However, in 1933 Henrik Sjögren, a Swedish ophthalmologist brought this fact into attention to the medical fraternity. In 1953, a paper by Morgan and Castleman explained the relationship between glandular involvement of salivary gland in Mikulicz's disease and Sjögren's disease wherein they suggested that both disease processes were either alike or part of the same disease with Mikulicz's disease being a milder form.[2]

It is now agreed that both Mikulicz'z disease and Sjögren's syndrome are closely related to each other and are autoimmune in origin; wherein the salivary tissue itself becomes antigenic.[2,45]

Clinical features

1. It behaves as an inflammatory as well as a neoplastic disease.[45]
2. It manifests as a diffuse, poorly outlined, unilateral or bilateral enlargement of the parotid or submandibular glands with an occasional increase or decrease in size of the swelling.
3. Patient complains of mild local discomfort, occasional pain and xerostomia.
4. Onset may be associated with fever, upper respiratory tract infection, tooth extraction or some other local inflammatory disorder.
5. Sometimes the lacrimal glands may be enlarged.
6. It occurs more frequently in the female population, particularly in the middle age or later.

Histopathology[45]

It shows orderly infiltrating lymphocytes which destroy and replace the acini, with persistence of islands of epithelial cells representing the remains of gland ducts. The lymphoid element is diffuse with occasional presence of germinal centers. The epithelium may consist of ducts showing cellular proliferation and loss of polarity or as the disease persists, solid nests or clumps of poorly defined epithelial cells called 'epimyoepithelial islands' will be evident. They occasionally form a syncytium. It is suggested that such islands are formed due to proliferation of both ductal cells and peripheral myoepithelial cells. Advanced lesions show deposition of eosinophilic, hyaline material in the epithelial islands.

It should be differentiated from chronic sialadenitis, papillary cystadenoma lymphomatosum and uveoparotitis. Also, malignant lymphoma shows a similar histologic appearance except that the epimyoepithelial islands are absent, lymphoid element is atypical and there is infiltration of interlobular septa by lymphoid tissue.

Management

Both, surgical excision as well as radiotherapy has been used. Mild cases once diagnosed do not warrant any treatment. In some cases, the swelling might regress spontaneously. Persistent cases can be managed by sialadenectomy. Radiation is no more preferred due to a likelihood of radiation – induced cancers.[45]

Sjögren's syndrome

Sjögren's syndrome is also referred to as Sicca syndrome or Goujerat-Sjögren's syndrome.[45] It is a chronic autoimmune disorder of the exocrine glands which affects predominantly, but not exclusively, the salivary and lacrimal glands, leading to dryness of mouth and eyes.[46] The disease may be confined to exocrine glands (glandular disease) or may involve multiple extraglandular sites (systemic involvement) and can even evolve into a lymphoid malignancy.[46] However, a fully developed case of Sjögren's syndrome consists of a triad of symptoms–keratoconjunctivitis sicca, xerostomia and a systemic disease, usually but not always rheumatoid arthritis.[2]

Sjögren's syndrome can manifest as primary or secondary Sjögren's syndrome. Primary Sjögren's syndrome also known as Sicca complex presents with only dry eyes and dry mouth. Secondary Sjögren's syndrome has in addition to the above features systemic manifestations such as systemic lupus erythematosus, polyarteritis nodosa, polymyositis or scleroderma and rheumatoid arthritis.[45]

Etiology

Various etiologies have been suggested viz genetic, hormonal, infectious and immunologic or it may be a combination of various factors.[45] Altered immunologic response is the most important intrinsic factor responsible for this disease according to most of the authorities. Bertram et al confirmed the presence of antisalivary duct antibodies in the serum of patients with Sjögren's syndrome in 75% of the cases.[45]

Clinical features

Females are predominantly affected. Age ranges from 5 years to 73 years, average being 50 years. Arthritis is the most frequent first complaint, followed by ocular complaints. Salivary gland symptoms are third in order of frequency.

Oral component

Xerostomia (dry mouth) is a predominant symptom resulting from decreased salivary secretion from both major and minor glands.[2] The common complaints are difficulty in chewing and swallowing, sore mouth, recurrent dental caries, typically cervical caries, due to increased plaque formation. Teeth may be hypocalcified. The oral mucosa is dry, sticky, erythematous and may have evidence of fungal infection. The tongue appears bald with loss of filiform papillae and fissuring of tongue.[46] Edentulous patients find it difficult to wear dentures.[2,46] Due to inadequate salivary secretions, retrograde infections further complicate the disease.[2]

Salivary flow rate studies to quantify the salivary gland function involve placement of collection cup over the duct orifice collection of stimulated secretion for a fixed time period. It usually shows diminished secretions. The saliva is usually cloudy due to pus and abnormally viscous due to gel-like consistency.[2] Occasionally, the saliva has a characteristic snowflake appearance caused by floculations of mucopus in a relatively clear aqueous background.[2] Parotid gland enlargement is seen in 25–66% cases of primary Sjögren's syndrome but is uncommon in secondary cases. Swellings may be recurrent and episodic, or chronic and fixed.

Ocular component

Xeropthalmia is another important manifestation of this condition. There is diminished tear production due to lymphocytic cell replacement of the lacrimal gland parenchyma.[2] This decreasing tear formation leads to chronic irritation and destruction of the corneal and bulbar conjunctival epithelium, referred to as Keratoconjunctivitis sicca.[46] The patient experiences redness, itchiness or burning sensation in the eye, rope-like secretions, dryness and a foreign body sensation in the eye and may not be able to tolerate smoke, air draft or light.[2,46]

On examination, bulbar conjunctival vessels are dilated, irregularity of the corneal image and occasionally enlargement of the lacrimal gland.[46] Schirmer's test can be performed to quantify the lacrimal secretions. Two 5 × 35 mm of red litmus paper strips are placed in the conjunctival sac area by light retraction of the lower eyelid. Moistening of the paper is measured after a period of 5 minutes. If there is less than 5 mm of moistening, the test is considered positive for decreased lacrimal secretions.[2] However, it is not diagnostic for keratoconjunctivitis sicca.[47]

Staining of the corneal and conjunctival epithelium by Rose Bengal dye is a more specific assay for diagnosis of kerato-conjunctivitis sicca.[46] Tear breakup time test evaluates the tear film integrity labeled by a drop of fluorescin. Overly rapid break-up of the film indicates abnormality of either the mucin or lipid layer of tears.[47]

Autoimmune manifestation

Rheumatoid arthritis is the most common autoimmune disorder associated with Sjögren's syndrome. At least half of the patients diagnosed with Sjögren's syndrome present with rheumatoid arthritis or develop it during the course of the disease.[2] High serum concentration of C – reactive protein are not usually detected in primary Sjögren's syndrome but may be seen in patients with rheumatoid arthritis and secondary Sjögren's syndrome.[46] In a study by Ericson et al, glandular abnormalities were found in many patients with rheumatoid arthritis without any glandular complaints. Also, salivary duct antibodies were found in 45% of patients.[2] Other autoimmune diseases associated with secondary Sjögren's syndrome include systemic lupus erythematosus (SLE), scleroderma, primary biliary cirrhosis.

Musculoskeletal manifestations

Patients complain of easy fatigue, general malaise, low-grade fever, myalgias and arthralgias. Muscle enzymes are usually within normal or mildly elevated and severe myositis is unusual.[46]

Respiratory tract involvement

The entire respiratory tract including the mediastinum and pleura may be mildly involved and may not have a clinical significance. Symptoms range from dry cough due to xerotrachea to dyspnoea due to interstitial disease or even airway obstruction.[48] High resolution CT scan shows bronchial and peribronchial thickening whereas transbronchial biopsies show bronchiolar lymphoid infiltrates and follicular bronchiolitis.[46]

Ear involvement

Sensorineural hearing loss is associated with Sjögren's syndrome in 21 to 46% of cases.[49,50] It is associated with high incidence of anticardiolipin antibody.[50]

Gastrointestinal and hepatobiliary manifestations

Dysphagia results from drying of pharynx and esophagus. Biopsy of gastric mucosa shows chronic atrophic gastritis and lymphocytic infiltrates. Patients have hypopepsinogenemia, elevated serum gastrin levels, low serum vitamin B_{12} levels and antibodies to parietal cells.[51] liver biopsy is suggestive of stage I primary biliary cirrhosis.[46] So also, sicca manifestations are seen in 50 % to 80% of patients with primary biliary cirrhosis.[52]

Urinary tract involvement

Urine acidification test is abnormal in one third of the patients with Sjögren's syndrome where as 10% patients manifest clinically with overt renal disease.[53] Interstitial disease is most common renal pathology. Patients present with distal tubular acidosis which may or may not be symptomatic.[46] Untreated renal tubular acidosis may lead to nephrocalcinosis, renal stones and compromised renal function.[54]

Vascular involvement

Raynaud's phenomenon is seen in more than one third of the patients with primary Sjögren's syndrome and may precede sicca manifestation. These patients may show soft tissue calcifications, but no digital ulcers and telangiectasia like scleroderma. Inflammatory vascular disease is reported in 20 to 30% cases of Sjögren's syndrome.[46]

Neuropsychiatric involvement

Neurologic involvement, mainly in the form of peripheral sensory or sensory-motor polyneuropathy or mononeuritis multiplex, occurs in 10 to 20% cases. Single nerve afflictions such as Carpal tunnel syndrome, sensory gangliopathies as well as cranial neuropathy have been described.[55] Anxiety, depressed mood and personality structure disorders are observed frequently and may be associated with deregulated stress response.[46]

Other manifestations

Varieties of cutaneous lesions are seen due to skin dryness, vasculitis and frequent allergic reactions. Clinically overt autoimmune thyroiditis has also been described. Mild normochromic, normocytic anemia is seen commonly. Elevated ESR is seen in 70% patients.[46]

Radiographic features

Sialography may be of diagnostic value in Sjögren's syndrome. Sialographs show formation of punctuate, cavitatory defcts which are filed with radiopaque contrast media. This sialographic presentation is referred to as 'cherry blossom appearance' or 'branchless fruit-laden tree appearance'.[45] Actually, the contrast medium extravasates through the weakened salivary gland ducts to produce the sialographic features. Poor elimination of contrast medium is seen.[45]

Histopathology

Patients with Sjögren's syndrome manifest destructive histo-pathologic lesions in one or more organs associated with focal or mononuclear cell infiltrates. These infiltrates contribute to the clinical manifestation of the disease. There is focal adenitis of the salivary, lacrimal and mucosal glands. In addition, there is atrophic gastritis, primary biliary cirrhosis, tubulointerstitial nephritis, interstitial pneumonitis, follicular bronchioloitis and vasculitis. Lymphocytic infiltrates are potentially progressive and may progress variably to B cell lymphoma.[46]

Salivary gland pathology is the most consistent feature of Sjögren's syndrome. Labial salivary gland biopsy is used as a means of assessment of salivary pathology in Sjögren's syndrome and can be used as a diagnostic test.[46,56]

Differential diagnosis

It includes other transient or chronic medical conditions responsible for keratoconjunctivitis sicca, xerostomia or parotid gland enlargement including infections, endocrinopathies and deficiency and degenerative disorders.[46]

Management

As Sjögren's syndrome is a chronic, potentially systemic disease of unknown etiology, treatment is largely empirical and symptomatic. Xerostomia and keratoconjunctivitis sicca are managed by use of artificial saliva and tears (0.5% methylcellulose) so that complications arising from these conditions can be prevented. Preventive dental care and fluoride application and maintenance of general hygiene is necessary. Patients should avoid environments with low humidity and also wear soft contact lenses.

Eye-patching and boric acid ointment can be used for corneal ulcers. Pilocarpine hydrochloride can be used as a secretagogue for management of xeropthalmia and xerostomia. Systemic cortico-steroids can be used for systemic complications such as vasculitis, glomerulonephritis and interstitial lung disease.

Cystic conditions

True cysts of the parotid gland constitute 2 to 5% of all parotid lesions. The cysts may be either acquired or congenital.[57] Type I branchial arch cysts are a duplication anomaly of the membranous external auditory canal whereas type II cysts are a duplication anomaly of the membranous and cartilaginous external auditory canal.[57] Excision during a quiescent period with preservation of facial nerve is curative.[57]

Mucoceles and mucous retention cysts almost invariably involve the minor salivary glands on the lips, buccal mucosa and ventral portion of the tongue.[57]

Mucoceles

Mucous retention cysts are true cysts with an epithelial lining and result from duct obstruction.[57] In contrast, mucoceles do not have an epithelial lining and are not true cysts. Infact, they represent a mucous extravasation into surrounding soft tissues following trauma to the glands.[57]

Etiopathogenesis

It arises from obstruction of the duct of a minor or accessory salivary gland. Traumatic severance of a salivary duct due to biting of lips, cheeks, tongue or due to injury due to lip pinching during extraction is the etiologic preceding factor. Even a chronic partial obstruction of the duct may lead to retention cyst. Up to 20% lesions may represent true retention cyst secondary to obstruction or microliths.[57]

However, majority of cases are an extravasation type of cysts which result from collection of salivary secretions in the soft tissues due to traumatic injury to the gland or duct.

Clinical features

The most common site is lower lips, cheek, tongue and floor of mouth **(Figure 7.10)**. Palatal minor salivary glands may also be involved with this condition.[58]

There is no sex predilection, occurring with same frequency in both males and females. It also occurs from birth to ninth decade, so any specific age predilection does not exist.

Non-neoplastic diseases 81

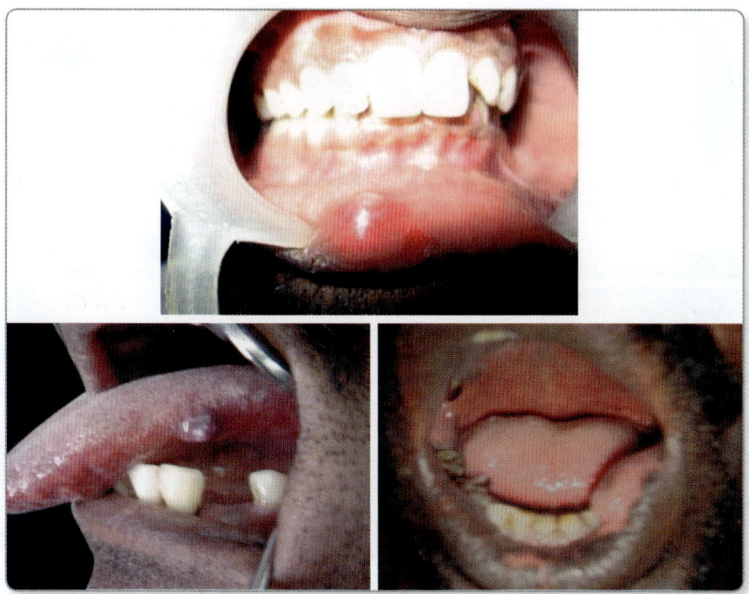

Figure 7.10 Mucoceles of the lower lip and tongue

It may be superficial or deep. Superficial lesions appear like a circumscribed, raised vesicle with a bluish translucent hue due to the thin overlying mucosa. However, deeper lesions being covered by normal mucosa have a normal color and texture.

Mucoceles over the lip and cheek once formed may get traumatized and rupture and the size decreases spontaneously. It enlarges again after a period of few days. Recurrence is usually common after spontaneous rupture.

Histopathology[58]

Majority of mucoceles are of extravasation type.[58] They consist of a circumscribed cavity in the connective tissue and submucosa producing an obvious elevation of the mucosa with thinning of the epithelium as though it is stretched. The cavity is not lined by epithelium. The wall is made up of lining of compressed fibrous connective tissue and fibroblasts. Commonly, the connective tissue wall is essentially granulation tissue, with infiltration of poly-morphonuclear leukocytes, lymphocytes and plasma cells.

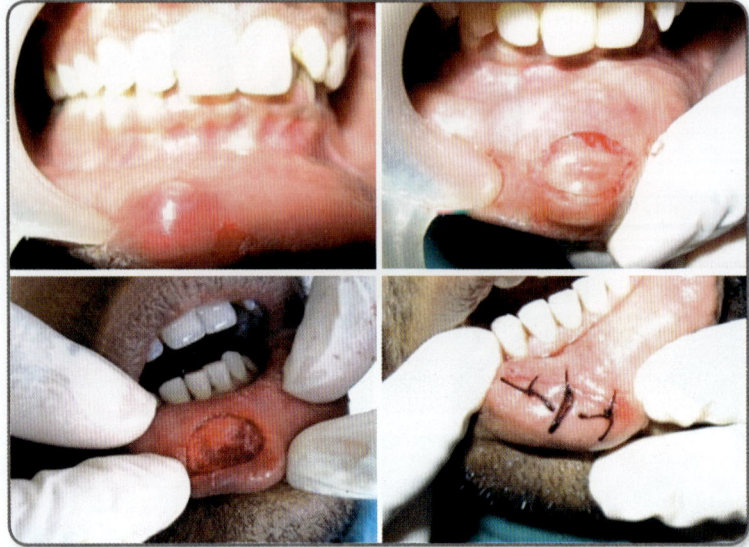

Figure 7.11 Management of mucocele over lip

Differential diagnosis[59]

Low-grade mucoepidermoid carcinoma, cavernous hemangioma, small lymphangioma and venous varix give a similar clinical appearance. Also, rarely a vascular leiomyoma appears blue and has a predilection for lip.

Management

Excision is the treatment of choice **(Figure 7.11)**. If the lesion is incised and drained, it gets filled up again as the incision heals. Along with the mucocele, a few normal minor salivary glands are also excised. Care should be taken to avoid creation of any other partially transsected minor salivary glands which might give rise to the recurrent mucocele.[59]

Ranula

Ranula is a form of mucocele which refers specifically to a mucocele arising in the floor of the mouth and is associated with the sublingual glands.[58] The etiopathogenesis essentially remains the same.

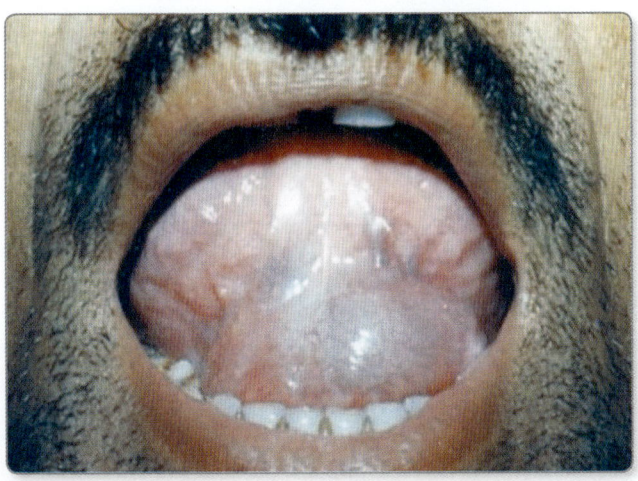

Figure 7.12 Ranula in the floor of the mouth (*Source:* Dr Suhas Jajoo)

Clinical features

It is slightly rare as compared to mucocele. They present as a slow growing, painless mass in the floor of the mouth.[58] Ranulas are usually large (3–6 cm) and form a blue, tense vesicle in the floor of the mouth **(Figure 7.12)**. The appearance is of that of a frog's belly and hence the term ranula (frog belongs to genus 'Rana').[59]

On palpation, it appears as a firm mass. If it is deep enough, the typical bluish color may not be evident.[59] The cyst is usually present above the mylohyoid curtain but then mylohyoid does not always from a complete diaphram and allows the leakage of the saliva below the mylohyoid allowing the lesion to present in the upper part of neck which is called as a "plunging ranula". Plunging ranulas may grow to a sufficient size so as to compromise respiration and swallowing and may also extend into mediastinum.[59]

Histopathology[58]

It is similar to the mucocele except that it sometimes shows a definite epithelial lining which is absent in the mucocele **(Figures 7.13A to C)**. Hence, it is considered by many investigators as a true retention cyst which occurs due to blockade of the duct.

Differential diagnosis[59]

If the ranula is deeper and the bluish color of swelling is not evident, a dermoid cyst may be considered in the differential diagnosis. A salivary

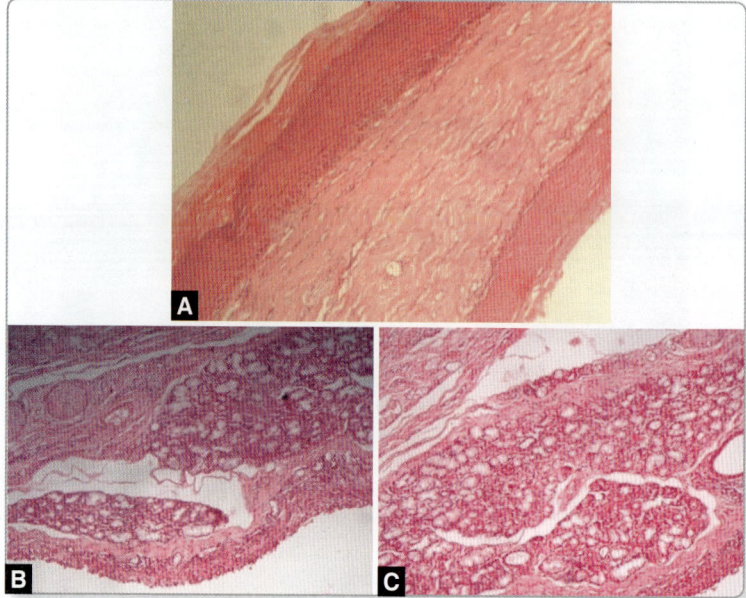

Figures 7.13A to C Histopathologic picture 10X magnification. (A) Mucous retention phenomenon; (B and C) Mucous extravasation phenomenon

gland tumor may also be considered in addition to a lymphangioma, lymph node enlargement suggestive of lymphoma, sarcoidosis or HIV related lymphadenopathy.

Management

Most predictable option is excision of the ranula and entire sublingual gland through a transoral approach. However, care should be taken to avoid damage to the lingual nerve. However, other modalities include deroofing of the ranula and marsupiali-zation. The ranula is deroofed and the mucosa sutured to the cystic lining followed by open packing of the cyst and sequentially reducing the size of the pack till it heals completely.

Salivary fistula

The injuries to the duct of the salivary gland lead to extravasation of the saliva in the soft tissue. The saliva fails to drain in the oral cavity. The injuries could be due to penetrating injuries on the check or as a result of the accidental damage during the surgical procedure. The saliva collects in

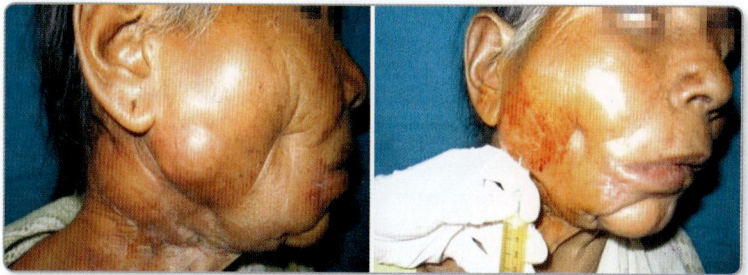

Figure 7.14 Sialocele following ablative tumor surgery

the adjoining soft tissue and produces asymptomatic swelling unless there is secondary infection. The collection of the saliva is the soft tissue plane is termed as sialocele. The swelling gradually erodes the overlying skin and forms a fistula, which drains saliva. The discharge is watery in nature and has a classical relation to the meals as it is aggravated during the meals. Secondary infection can set in and in such event the condition becomes symptomatic and the discharge becomes purulent in nature. Depending on the nature of the duct that is damaged the salivary fistula can be labeled as major or minor fistula. If the main duct is damaged, the major fistula is formed and if the small collecting duct is severed then the minor salivary fistula results.

The management of this condition comprises the following:

1. *Conservative management:* It is generally done for the minor fistulas. A compression dressing is given which prevents the cutaneous drainage of the saliva, and the mounting pressure of saliva within the tissue finds a way out in the oral cavity through the transected distal end of the duct. The pressure is maintained till the tract is formed between the two severed ends of the duct. The minor salivary fistulas close with the conservative treatment and the cutaneous drainage of the saliva stops spontaneously.
2. *Anastomosis of the severed duct:* If the fistula is of recent onset then the area is explored surgically and the two severed ends are identified and anastomosed over the PVC canula **(Figure 7.15)**. Ideally, silicone tubing is used for cannulation, but a PVC tube also does the job satisfactorily.
3. Total excision of the involved gland in case of the persistent major fistula which fails to respond to conservative treatment and where the anastomosis of the duct is not possible due to loss of tissue, the involved gland may be excised.
4. *Irradiation of the gland:* Irradiation renders the gland fibrotic and non functional and the fistula gets obliterated.

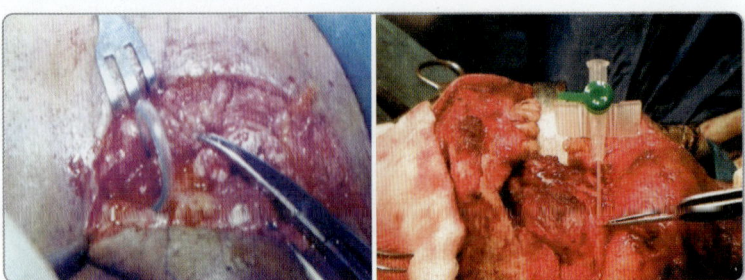

Figure 7.15 Cannulation of duct with PVC tube

References

1. McQuone SJ. Acute viral and bacterial infections of the salivary glands. Rice DH, Eisele DW, (Eds). Otolaryngol Clin N Am. 1999;32(5):793- 811.
2. Mandel L. Inflammatory disorders – Clinicopathologic considerations. Diseases of Salivary glands. Rankow RM, Polayes IM (Eds). WB Saunders, Philadelphia. 1976;9(1):202-38.
3. Raad II, Sabbagh MF, Caransos GJ. Acute bacterial sialadenitis: A study of 29 cases and review. Rev Infect Dis. 1990;12:591 – 601.
4. Petersdorf RG, Forsyth BR, Bernanke D. Staphylococcal parotitis. N Engl J Med. 1958;259:1250-58.
5. Seifert G. Etiology and histological classification of sialadenitis. Pathologica. 1997;89:7-17.
6. Tabak LA, Levine MJ, Mandel ID. Role of salivary mucins in the protection of oral cavity. J Oral Pathol. 1982;11:1-17.
7. Rousseau P. Acute suppurative parotitis. J Am Geriatr Soc. 1990;38:897- 98.
8. McAdams RM, Mair EA, Rajnik M. Neonatal suppurative submandibular sialadenitis: case report and literature review. Int J Pediatr Otorhinolaryngol. 2005;69:993-7.
9. Brook I. Suppurative sialadenitis associated with anaerobic bacteria in newborns. Pediatr Infect Dis J. 2006;25:280.
10. Brook I. The bacteriology of salivary gland infections. Turner MD, Glickman R. (Eds). Oral Maxillofac Surg Clin N Am. 2009;21:269-74.
11. Lewis MAO, Lamey PJ, Gibson J. Quantitative bacteriology of a case of acute parotitis. Oral Surg Oral Med Oral Pathol. 1989;68:571-75.
12. Carlson ER. Diagnosis and management of salivary gland infections. Turner MD, Glickman R. (Eds). Oral Maxillofac Surg Clin N Am. 2009;21:293-312.
13. Carlson ER, Ord RA. Infections of the salivary glands. In Carlson ER, Ord RA, (Eds). Textbook and color atlas of salivary gland pathology. Diagnosis and management. Ames (IA): Wiley Blackwell; 2008:67- 89.

14. Brook I. Diagnosis and management of parotitis. Arch Otolaryngol Head Neck Surg. 1992;118:469-71.
15. Guardia SN, Cameron R, Phillips A. Fatal necrotizing mediastinitis secondary to acute suppurative parotitis. J Otolaryngol. 1991;20:54-6.
16. Pang YT, Raine CH. Acute suppurative parotitis and facial paralysis. J Laryngol Otol. 1996;110:91-2.
17. Andrews JC, Abemayor E, Alessi DM. Parotitis and facial nerve dysfunction. Arch Otolaryngol Head Neck Surg. 1989;115:240-2.
18. Rice DH. Chronic inflammatory disorders of the salivary glands. Rice DH, Eisele DW, (Eds). Salivary gland disorders. Otolaryngol Clin N Am. 1999; 32(5): 813-8.
19. Nahlieli O, Bar T, Shacham R. Management of chronic recurrent parotitis: current therapy. J Oral Maxillofac Surg. 2004;62:1150-55.
20. Baurmash HD. Chronic recurrent parotitis: A closer look at its origin, diagnosis and management. J Oral Maxillofac Surg. 2004;62:1010-18.
21. Batsakis GJ, Sylvest V. Pathology of Salivary glands. Chicago. American society of Clinical Pathologists. 1977
22. http://www.eaom.net/app/prvt/VediNotizia.d/Notizia-89. Accessed 02/10/2009 @ 1.10pm IST
23. Turner MD. Sialoendoscopy and salivary gland sparing surgery. Turner MD, Glickman R (Eds). Oral Maxillofac Surg Clin N Am. 2009;21:323-9.
24. Williams MF. Sialolithiasis. Rice DH, Eisele DW, (Eds). Salivary gland disorders. Otolaryngol Clin N Am. 1999;32(5):819-34.
25. Harrison JD, Epivatianos A, Bhatia SN. Role of microliths in the etiology of chronic submandibular sialadenitis: A clinicopathological investigation of 154 cases. Histopathology 1997;31:237-51.
26. Arrieta AJ, McCaffrey TV. Inflammatory disorders of Salivary glands. In: Cummins Otolaryngology – Head and Neck Surgery, Mosby; 4th edn. 2005; 58(5):1323-38.
27. Work WP, Hecht DW. Inflammatory diseases of the major salivary glands. In: Papparella MM, Shumrick DF (Eds). Otolaryngology, Philadelphia, WB Saunders. 1980;3:2235-43.
28. Lustmann J, Regev E, Melamed Y. Sialolithiasis: A survey on 245 patients and a review of literature. Int J Oral Maxillofac Surg. 1990;19:135-8.
29. Berini-Aytes L, Gay-Escoda C. Morbidity associated with removal of the submandibular gland. J craniomaxillofac Surg. 1992;20:216-9.
30. Ellies M, Laskawi R, Arglebe C. Surgical management of non-neoplastic diseases of the submandibular gland. A follow-up study. Int J Oral Maxillofac Surg. 1996;25:285-9.
31. Rice DH. Diseases of the Salivary Glands – non-neoplastic. In: Bailey BJ, Johnson JT, Kohut RI. (Eds). Head and Neck Surgery – Otolaryngology; Philadelphia, JB Lipincott 1993;1:475-84.

32. Baurmash H, Dechiara S. Extraoral parotid sialolithotomy. J Oral Maxillofac Surg. 1991;49:127-32.
33. Iro H, Waitz G, Nitsche N. Extracorporeal piezoelectric shock-wave lithotripsy of salivary gland stones. Laryngoscope. 1992;102:492-4.
34. Iro H, Zenk J, Waldfahrer F. Extracorporeal shock wave lithotripsy of parotid stones results of a prospective clinical trial. Ann Otol Rhinol Laryngol. 1998;107:860-4.
35. Ottaviani F, Capaccio P, Campi M. Extracorporeal electromagnetic shock-wave lithotripsy for salivary gland stones. Laryngoscope 1996;106:761-4.
36. McAnnally T. Parotitis: Clinical presentations and management. Postgrad Med. 1982;71:87-99.
37. Rice DH. Salivary gland disorders: Neoplastic and Non-neoplastic. Med Clin North Am. 1999;83(1):197 – 217.
38. Brunell PA, Brickman A, Steinberg S. Parotitis in children who had previously received mumps vaccine. Pediatrics. 1972;50:441-4.
39. Shafer WG, Hine MK, Levy BM. Bacterial, Viral and Mycotic infections. A textbook of Oral Pathology. Harcourt Asia PTE Ltd. Singapore. 4th edn. 1993;6:340-405.
40. Peltola H, Kulkarni P. Mumps outbreaks in Canada and the United states: Time for new thinking on Mumps vaccines. Clin Infect Dis. 2007;45:459- 66.
41. Shanti RM, Aziz SR. HIV – associated Salivary gland disease. Turner MD, Glickman R. (Eds). Oral Maxillofac Surg Clin N Am. 2009;21:339-43.
42. Capaccio P, Monforte A, Moroni M. Salivary stone lithotripsy in the HIV patient. Oral Surg Oral Med Oral Radiol Endod. 2002;93(5):552-4.
43. Morales-Aguirre JJ, Patino-Nino AP, Mendoza-Aspiri M. Parotid cysts in children infected with human immunodeficiency virus. Arch Otolaryngol Head Neck Surg. 2005;131:353-5.
44. Schiodt M, Dodd C, Greenspan D. Natural history of HIV-associated salivary gland disease. Oral Surg Oral Med Oral Pathol. 1992;74:327
45. Shafer WG, Hine MK, Levy BM. Tumors of salivary glands. A textbook of Oral Pathology. Harcourt Asia PTE Ltd. Singapore. 4th edn 1993;3:231-57.
46. Manoussakis MN, Moutsopoulos HM. Sjögren's syndrome. Rice DH, Eisele DW, (Eds). Otolaryngol Clin N Am. 1999;32(5):843-60.
47. Kincaid MC. The eye in Sjögren's syndrome. In: Talal N, Moutsopoulos HM, Kasan SS (Eds). Sjögren's syndrome: Clinical and immunological aspects. Berlin, Springer-Verlag. 1987.p.25
48. Constantopoulos SH, Moutsopoulos HM. The Respiratory system in Sjögren's syndrome. In: Talal N, Moutsopoulos HM, Kasan SS (Eds). Sjögren's syndrome: Clinical and immunological aspects. Berlin, Springer-Verlag. 1987.p.83.
49. Trott MS, Hughes GB, Calabrese LH. Hearing and Sjögren's syndrome. Ear Nose Throat J. 1996;75:666.
50. Tumiati B, Casoli P, Parmeggiani A. Hearing loss in Sjögren's syndrome. Ann Intern Med. 1997;126:450.

51. Trevino H, Tsianos EB, Schenker S. Gastrointestinal and hepatobiliary features in Sjögren's syndrome. In: Talal N, Moutsopoulos HM, Kasan SS (Eds). Sjögren's syndrome: Clinical and immunological aspects. Berlin, Springer-Verlag. 1987:pg.83.
52. Tsianos EV, Hoofnagle JH, Fox PC. Sjögren's syndrome in patients with primary biliary cirrhosis. Hepatology. 1990;11:730.
53. Kassan SS, Talal N. Renal disease with Sjögren's syndrome. In: Talal N, Moutsopoulos HM, Kasan SS (Eds). Sjögren's syndrome: Clinical and immunological aspects. Berlin, Springer-Verlag. 1987.p.96.
54. Moutsopoulos HM, Cledes J, Skopouli FN. Nephrocalcinosis in Sjögren's syndrome. J Int Med. 1991;230:187.
55. Alexander El. Neuromuscular complications of primary Sjögren's syndrome. In: Talal N, Moutsopoulos HM, Kasan SS (Eds). Sjögren's syndrome: Clinical and immunological aspects. Berlin, Springer-Verlag. 1987.p.61.
56. Daniels TE, Aufdermorte TB, Greenspan JS. Histopathology of Sjögren's syndrome. In: Talal N, Moutsopoulos HM, Kasan SS (Eds). Sjögren's syndrome: Clinical and immunological aspects. Berlin, Springer-Verlag. 1987.p.61.
57. Rice DH. Salivary gland disorders: Neoplastic and Non-neoplastic. Med Clin N Am. 1999;83(1):197-217.
58. Shafer WG, Hine MK, Levy BM. Physical and chemical injuries of the oral cavity. A textbook of Oral Pathology. Harcourt Asia PTE Ltd. Singapore. 4th edn. 1993;10:528-93.
59. Marx DE, Stern D. Non-neoplastic salivary gland disease. In: Oral and maxillofacial pathology: A rationale for diagnosis and treatment. Quintessence publishing co, Inc. New Delhi. 2003;11:497-527.

Etiology and pathogenesis of tumors

chapter 8

The etiology of salivary gland tumors is unknown. However investigations have been carried out to link salivary gland neoplasms to etiologic factors like viruses, radiation, occupation, lifestyle, hormones, etc.

1. *Viruses:* Epstein-Barr viruses have been implicated in the etiology of malignant lymphoepithelial lesion, a form of malignant salivary gland carcinoma.[1] This tumor is very rare in people who are not of Asian extraction. Merrick and colleagues believe that environmental factors in Greenland Eskimo children enhance humoral immunity to Epstein-Barr virus, because 100% of children are primarily infected with the virus. The virus is present in the pharynx and salivary glands of this population. Hence the interrelationships of immunity, environmental factors and genetic constitution of the host may all play a role in malignant transformation of salivary gland epithelial cells. The other viruses suspected as possible etiologic agents are polyoma virus, cytomegalovirus, type C particles similar to those associated with murine leukemia, type B particles similar to those associated with murine breast tumors and human papilloma virus types 16 and 18.

2. *Radiation:* Evidence exists for the relationship between exposure to ionizing radiation and the later development of salivary gland tumors.[1] The tumorigenic effect of therapeutic radiation of head and neck on salivary glands has been assessed thoroughly. The minimum tumorigenic effect is difficult to estimate and remains controversial. The substantial lymphoid component of the parotid gland may be more susceptible to low-dose radiation damage than the parenchyma. A dose of 483 rad measured one centimeter below the skin in the parotid gland appears to significantly increase the risk of tumor development.[1] In many cases it is difficult to determine if the glands were exposed to the primary beam or the scattered rays. It seems that doses as low as 140 rad may increase the risk of developing salivary gland neoplasms. Patients with radiation-related salivary gland tumors experience a high rate of second tumors of salivary, thyroid and parathyroid glands. Parotid gland is the site of radiation-associated neoplasm in most of the reported cases. Radiation induced salivary gland neoplasms follow a pattern similar to those found in the thyroid gland with latent periods ranging from 15 to 20 years. Most common tumor seen in this group was benign mixed tumor in one study and in another study there was an increased incidence of mucoepidermoid and epidermoid carcinomas.[2] Ultraviolet

radiation may also be associated with an increased risk of salivary gland cancer.[3]
3. *Occupation:* People in occupations such as asbestos mining, manufacturing of rubber products leading to increased exposure to nitrosamines, industries that use these rubber products such as shoe manufacturing, plumbing (exposure to metals) and woodworking in the automobile industry are more prone to develop salivary gland carcinoma.[1] Similarly people associated with an increased exposure to silica dust are more prone to salivary gland tumors.
4. *Lifestyle:* Researchers could demonstrate no association of salivary gland tumors with heavy smoking or heavy alcohol consumption.[4] However, cigarette smoking may play a causative role in the development of epidermoid carcinomas.[5] Warthin's tumor is strongly associated with cigarette smoking.[6] Although severe malnutrition such as kwashiorkor causes enlargement of salivary glands, increased incidence of salivary gland tumors have not been observed.
5. *Endogenous hormones* may have a role in carcinogenesis of salivary gland tumors. Studies have indicated the presence of estrogen receptors in 80% of normal salivary glands and prolactin-binding activity in both normal and neoplastic salivary gland tissue.
6. There has been an increased incidence of salivary gland tumors in patients with breast cancer.[7,8]

Tobacco and alcohol, which are highly associated with head neck squamous cell carcinoma, have not been shown to play a role in the development of malignancies of the salivary glands. However tobacco smoking has been associated with the development of Warthin tumors (papillary cystadenoma lymphomatosum). Although smoking is highly associated with head and neck squamous cell carcinoma, it does not appear to be associated with salivary gland malignancies.

The etiology of salivary gland neoplasms is not fully understood. Two theories predominate: The bicellular stem cell theory and the multicellular theory.[9]

Bicellular stem cell theory[9]

This theory holds that tumors arise from 1 of 2 undifferentiated stem cells viz: the excretory duct reserve cell or the intercalated duct reserve cell. Excretory stem cells give rise to squamous cell and mucoepidermoid carcinomas, while intercalated stem cells give rise to pleomorphic adenomas, oncocytomas, adenoid cystic carcinomas, adenocarcinomas, and acinic cell carcinomas.

Multicellular theory[9]

In the multicellular theory, each tumor type is associated with a specific differentiated cell of origin within the salivary gland unit. Squamous cell carcinomas arise from excretory duct cells, pleomorphic adenomas arise from the intercalated duct cells, oncocytomas arise from the striated duct cells, and acinic cell carcinomas arise from acinar cells.

Pathophysiology of salivary gland tumors

Although molecular events that lead to the formation of salivary gland neoplasms are not well understood, more substantial observations and correlations have been discovered and published.

Many studies have investigated the role that tumor suppressor genes, especially the p53 family, play in the development of salivary gland neoplasms. One study found p53 mutations to be important in the development of both benign and malignant salivary gland neoplasms and that most mutations occurred in the fifth and eighth exons of the gene. Benign salivary neoplasms, pleomorphic adenomas, myoepitheliomas, and basal cell adenomas expressed increased levels of transactivation-incompetent truncated isoforms of p63 and p73, while lower levels of normal forms have been found in normal salivary tissue. Further inquiry found the delta np73l isoform of p63 was expressed in tumors and not healthy salivary gland tissue. Overexpression of p53 has been identified in a high percentage of carcinomas that arise from pleomorphic adenomas.

The function of oncogenes is also being elucidated. Murine double minute 2 (MDM2), a cellular protooncogene, which is capable, if amplified, of causing tumorigenesis by inactivating the p53 tumor-suppressor gene, has been found to be overexpressed in varying types of benign and malignant salivary gland tumors overexpressed in varying types of benign and malignant salivary gland tumors. Over expression of MDM2 along with high–mobility group protein gene (HMGIC) has also been shown to lead to malignant changes that cause carcinoma expleomorphic adenoma. Mutated K-ras has been shown in mouse models to activate cellular pathways that lead to increased truncated p63 expression that inhibits p53 transcriptional activity.

Studies that look at the neovascularization in salivary gland neoplasms have revealed factors that increase angiogenesis and are important in the development of salivary gland neoplasms. High levels of nitric oxide synthase and vascular endothelial growth factor (VEGF) correlate with clinical stage, tumor size, vascular invasion, recurrence, metastases, poorer prognogen, and increased aggressiveness in salivary gland neoplasms. The role of nitrogen oxide is also beginning to be investigated in the tumorigenesis of warthin tumor.

Pleomorphic adenomas have been shown to have a high incidence of allelic loss on band 12q 13-15, HMGIC is a transcriptional activator located in this region, and recurrent translocations that involve this gene in benign

Etiology and pathogenesis of tumors 93

solid tumors, including pleomorphic adenomas, have been discovered. High mobility groups AT-hook 1 (HMGIY) on band 6p21 rearrangements have been found to be closely associated with 12q translocations. However, pleomorphic adenomas have recently been found to be the only exception.

Additionally, recurrent translocations that involve PLAG1, a zinc finger gene located on band 8q 12, have been reported in pleomorphic adenomas. New evidence suggests that the effects of these translocations can occur without gross rearrangements but with gene overexpression due to radiation exposure. Overexpression of PLAG1 is correlated with overexpressed with other cancers, such as colorectal cancer and melanomas.

Other salivary gland neoplasms have been associated with overexpressed betacatenin through abnormal WNT signaling. Adenoid cystic carcinoma with mutations in CTNNM1 (b-catenin gene), AXIN1 (axis inhibition protein 1) and APC (adenomatosis polyposis coli tumor suppressor) shows tumorigenesis via this process. Promoter methylation is known to develop tumors by inactivating tumor suppressor genes. Mutations that cause hypermethylation and downregulation of 14-3-30, a target gene for p53 in the Gap2/mitosis (G2/M) cell cycle checkpoint, were found to be extensive in adenoid cystic carcinoma (ACC). The methylation of genes that control apoptosis and DNA repair were also found in ACC, especially in high grade tumors.

Chromosomal loss has been found to be an important cause of mutations and tumor genesis in salivary gland tumors. Allelic loss of chromosomal arm 19q has been reported to occur commonly in adenoid cystic carcinoma. Mucoepidermoid carcinomas also show the loss of chromosomal arms 2q.gp.12p. and 16q more than 50% of the time.

Multiple other genes are being investigated in the tumor genesis of salivary gland neoplasms hepatocyte growth factor (HGF), a protein that causes morphogenesis and dispersion of epithelial cells, has been found to increase adenoid cystic carcinoma scattering and perhaps invasiveness. Expression of proliferating cell nuclear antigen (PCNA) was found in the 2 most common malignant salivary tumors, mucoepidermoid carcinomas and adenoid cystic carcinomas. Overexpression of fibroblast growth factor 8b has been shown to lead to salivary gland tumors in transgenic mice.

New research in salivary gland neoplasms focuses on factors that increase tumor invasion and spread. Matrix metalloproteinase-1, tenascin-c, and beta-6 integrin have been found to be associated with benign tumor expansion and tissue invasion by malignant tumors. In adenoid cystic carcinoma, increased immunoreactivity for nerve growth and tyrosine kinase has been correlated with perineural invasion.

References

1. Spitz MR, Batsakis JG. Major salivary gland carcinoma. Arch Otolaryngol. 1984;110:45.
2. Hanna EY, Suen JY. Malignant tumors of the salivary glands. Myers EN, Suen JY, Myers JN, Hanna EY, Editors. Cancer of the head and neck. Saunders 4(21):475-510.
3. Stenman G, Mark J. Specificity of the involvement of chromosomes 8 and 12 in human mixed salivary-gland tumors. J Oral Pathol. 1983;12:446.
4. Auclair PL, Ellis GL, Douglas GR, Wenig BM, Janney CG. Salivary gland neoplasms: General considerations. Ellis GL, Editor. Surgical pathology of the salivary glands. WB Saunders, Philadelphia 1991;9:135-64.
5. Pinkston JA, Cole P. Cigarette smoking and Warthin's tumor. Am J Epidemiol. 1996;144:183-7.
6. Batsakis JG, Regezi JA. The pathology of head and neck tumors: Salivary glands, Part 1. Head Neck Surg. 1978;1:59.
7. Puterman M, Goldstein J. Primary lymph node Kaposi's sarcoma of the parotid gland. Head Neck Surg. 1983;5:535.
8. Baker SR, Malone B. Salivary gland malignancies in children. Cancer. 1985; 55:1730-6.
9. Califano J, Eisele DW. Benign salivary gland neoplasms. Rice DH, Eisele DW, Editors. Otolaryngol Clin N Am. 1999;32(5):861-74.

Incidence of salivary gland neoplasms

chapter 9

In most parts of the world the incidence of salivary gland tumors, both benign and malignant, varies from 1 to 2 per 100,000 populations per year.[1] Because of the rarity of tumors of the salivary glands, they are often included as "miscellaneous" or "other" head and neck tumors in epidemiologic surveys of neoplasia. The annual incidence of salivary gland tumors varies around the world from approximately 0.4 to 13.5 cases per 100,000 people.[2]

Salivary gland neoplasms do not exhibit any strong predilection for a particular sex nor is there any distinct racial incidence pattern. Patients of all ages can be affected.[3] However, the majority of salivary gland tumors are diagnosed between fourth and seventh decade.

Historically, an exception to the low incidence of salivary gland neoplasms is its incidence in Inuit population living in the western and central Canadian Artic. From 1950 to 1966 salivary gland neoplasms, predominantly Lymphoepithelial carcinoma accounted for approximately 25% of all cancers affecting this population. These tumors were so prevalent that the term 'Eskimomas' was coined to denote them. The mortality rate arising from these tumors was 100 and 400 times greater among Inuit men and women respectively as compared to Canadian men and women.[2]

In the United States, data on Salivary gland tumors is limited to incidence of salivary gland carcinomas. In 1959, Dorn and Cutler reported a higher incidence of salivary gland carcinoma in nonwhites than whites. Recent data (May 1989) from Surveillance, Epidemiology and End results (SEER) registries of the National Cancer Institute show the age-adjusted incidence of salivary gland cancer from 1982–1986 in all races and both sexes to be 0.9 cases per 100,000 people. Since malignant tumors comprise between 35 and 40% of all salivary gland tumors, it is estimated that annual incidence of salivary gland tumors in the United States is between 2.2 and 2.5 cases per 100,000 people.[2] It accounts for 650 deaths per year in the USA. In USA 3 - 4% of all neoplasms of the Head and Neck are salivary gland neoplasms. In UK it comprises of 40 cases per year.

AT CRI, Varanasi; 1 - 4 new cases per year are diagnosed as salivary gland tumors. They account for less than 1% of all registered malignancies.[3]

Following table gives the incidence of salivary gland tumors according to site:

Incidence of salivary gland tumors according to site[4]

	Parotid (%)	Submandibular (%)	Sublingual (%)	Minor glands[5] (Palate) (%)
Benign	80	60	30	53
Malignant	20	40	70	47

Age and sex predilection for major salivary gland tumors is as follows: Benign: 40 years and Malignant: 55 years.

Male predominance is seen in Warthin's tumor and female predominance in Acinic cell tumors.

Site and distribution[6]

Site	Distribution (%)	Malignant (%)
Parotid	75-80	17-20
Submandibular	5-10	50
Sublingual	1-2	80
Minor glands	10-20	50

References

1. I Van Der Waal. Salivary gland neoplasms. I Van Der Waal, Prabhu SR, Wilson DF, Daftary DK, Johnson NW, Editors. Oral diseases in the Tropics, Oxford University Press, Delhi 1993;41:478-86.
2. Spitz MR, Batsakis JG. Major salivary gland carcinoma. Arch Otolaryngol. 1984;110:45.
3. Sharma D. Salivary gland tumours. Text of Smt. Radha Devi Memorial Oration delivered on 29th December, 99 at Madurai during ASICON. Indian association of surgical oncology. (www.indiandoctors.com/iaso/htm. Accessed on 18th July,05)
4. Eneroth CM. Salivary gland tumors in the parotid gland, submandibular gland and the palate region. Cancer. 1971;27:1415-8.
5. Walker NI, Gobe GC. Cell death and cell proliferation during atrophy of the rat parotid gland induced by duct obstruction. J Pathol. 1987;152:333-44.
6. Cornog JL, Gray SR. Surgical and clinical pathology of salivary gland tumors. Rankow RM, Polayes IM, Editors. Diseases of Salivary glands. WB Saunders, Philadelphia. 1976;5:99-142.

Histogenesis of salivary gland neoplasms

chapter 10

Of all the tissues in the human body, perhaps the salivary glands have the most histologically heterogenous group of tumors and the greatest diversity of morphologic features among their cells and tissues. Classification of neoplasms of any organ should be predicated on patterns of differentiation that reflect the organization and cell types of the parental tissue. There is need to investigate various developmental processes, cell types, and the forms of differentiation involved in salivary gland tumors and to produce an improved criteria for the segregation of individual types of tumors.

Histogenetic concepts[1]

A variety of concepts for salivary gland tumors have evolved but the concept usually cited as central to the induction of these tumors is the semipluripotential bicellular reserve cell hypothesis. It is generally accepted that specific reserve or basal cells of the excretory and intercalated ducts or both are responsible for replacement of all types of cells in the normal gland and hence are the sole source for neoplastic transformation. Walker and Gobe have clearly shown that cells in the striated and intercalated ducts are capable of DNA synthesis on both the ligated and unligated sides and that the main cells dividing on the unligated side are striated duct and acinar cells. Such findings negate the reserve cell hypothesis.[2] However, as illustrated by certain tumors and morphologic concepts, there likely are basic structural patterns in the developing and mature salivary gland that are reflected in salivary gland tumors in general and in the various differentiation patterns within anyone subgroup specifically. The importance of this concept is that it relates the histology of neoplastic processes directly to the classification of salivary gland tumors.

It is generally accepted that the basal cells of the excretory duct and intercalated duct cells act as reserve cells for the more differentiated cells of the salivary gland unit, both during the later stages of development and in the mature gland. The basal cells of the excretory duct give rise to the columnar and squamous cells of the excretory duct and the intercalated duct cells give rise to the acinar cells, other intercalated duct cells, striated duct cells, and probably the myoepithelial cells. The importance of these two cells as reserve or progenitor cells in salivary gland development as well as tumor formation has been previously emphasized. Current classifications of neoplasms are based upon the ability of the neoplastic cell to mimic morphologically and functionally its cell of origin.

When this principle is applied to salivary gland neoplasms, two hypothetical possibilities are suggested. The first would be the genesis of neoplasms from their adult differentiated counterparts of the salivary gland unit. Under this scheme the acinous cell carcinomas would originate from acinar cells, oncocytic tumors from striated duct cells, squamous cell carcinomas and mucoepidermoid carcinomas from excretory duct cells and all other adenomas and adenocarcinomas from intercalated duct cells.

Second hypothetical possibility is more-plausible since it would not require dedifferentiation of already, highly specialized cells such as acinar and striated duct cells. Neoplasms under this scheme would generate from the two undifferentiated reserve cells discussed previously, the excretory duct reserve cell and the intercalated duct reserve cell. This bicellular theory of origin is similar to one previously proposed which was based on light microscopic findings only. Electron microscopic studies can now be added to light microscopic findings in support of this bicellular theory of salivary gland tumor histogenesis.

Batsakis theory of origin of salivary gland neoplasms is in agreement with Pierce's concept of development of general neoplasia i.e. pathology of the cells involved in tissue renewal. The genome of the normal cell contains all the information necessary for expression of normal as well as malignant phenotype. Malignancy is superimposed upon the process of cell renewal. Malignant stem cells are derived from normal stem cells by a process equivalent to post embryonic differentiation. If the stem cells capable of synthesizing DNA are oncogenic targets, malignancy results. If well differentiated cells still capable of one more differentiation are the oncogenic targets, a benign tumor results. Thus the stage of differentiation of the target cells decides whether the tumor is benign or malignant. Malignant tumor cells' capacity for proliferation and differentiation operate on a different level of control than the normal phenotypic expression.

Mixed tumor

Two main types of cells viz epithelial cells and myoepithelial cells have been described in mixed tumors. Other cells such as mesenchymal cells and indeterminate cells have also been reported. Hubner and associates have postulated that the myoepithelial cell is responsible for the morphologic diversity of the tumor including the production of fibrous, mucinous, chondroid and osseous areas. Regezi and Batsakis have postulated that intercalated duct reserve cell can differentiate into ductal and myoepithelial cells and the latter can undergo mesenchymal metaplasia since they have smooth muscle like properties. Dardick and associates state that neoplastically altered epithelial cell with a potential for multidirectional differentiation may be histogenetically responsible for the pleomorphic adenoma.[3] The epithelial cells, which vary from intercalated duct-like cells to epider-moid cells, comprise the histological majority of most tumors. Myoepithelial and myoepithelial like cells have been described in varying numbers, depending upon the tumor studied. These cells are most commonly found in the myxoid areas of mixed tumors.

Mixed tumors represent a spectrum of lesions dependent upon the relative number of epithelial and myoepithelial cells present. At one end of the spectrum would be monomorphic adenomas that would be composed primarily of epithelial cells, and at the other end of the spectrum would be myoepitheliomas composed primarily of myoepithelial cells. In the range between these two extremes would be the mixed tumors, composed of different ratios of epithelial and myoepithelial cells.

Adenoid cystic carcinoma

The morphological resemblance of adenoid cystic carcinoma cells to intercalated duct cells in both light and electron microscopic examinations have been accepted by researchers. The tumor cells are generally unremarkable and contain relatively few organelles. An inconsistently reported finding has been the presence of myoepithelial and myoepithelial-like cells, suggesting to some that this is the cell of origin of the adenoid cystic carcinoma. This apparent mixture of cells would seem analogous to the mixture seen in the mixed tumor, even though it is quantitatively different. The bicellular theory of origin would account for the appearance of both ductal and myoepithelial cells through neoplastic transformation of the intercalated duct reserve cell. On occasion the adenoid cystic carcinoma (microscopically) resembles the mixed tumor.

Squamous cell carcinoma and mucoepidermoid carcinoma

Theoretically all cells of the salivary gland unit carry the potential to keratinize or become squamous in type under appropriate circumstances because of their origin from surface epithelium.

The cells of the excretory duct would be expected to have the greatest potential for this phenomenon because of their lack of specialization and their proximity to the gland orifice. Reactive glandular changes, associated with such stimuli as smoking or infection, result in squamous metaplasia and occasionally mucous metaplasia of the excretory ducts.

Neoplastic transformation of such metaplastic excretory ducts may result in squamous cell carcinomas or mucoepidermoid carcinomas. Alternatively, either neoplasm can arise from direct neoplastic transformation of the excretory duct reserve cell, since this cell normally differentiates into squamous, columnar and mucous cells of the excretory duct. A squamous cell carcinoma would result if only squamous cells were produced. A low-grade mucoepidermoid carcinoma would result if differentiation was directed more toward the production of mucous cells than squamous, and a high-grade mucoepidermoid carcinoma would result if squamous cells were favored over mucous cells. Additional sup-port for the excretory duct reserve cell as the cell of origin comes from the observation by Eversole that mucoepidermoid carcinomas do not occur as intralobular lesions.

Oncocytic tumors

Oncocytes are cells that contain hyperplastic and pleomorphic mitochondria. These cells are generally not present in the salivary glands of younger individuals, but are commonly seen with increasing age. They may be found anywhere along the salivary gland unit, but are most frequently encountered among the intercalated duct cells and acinar cells. Oncocytes are believed to represent a form of cellular degeneration, since they lack the differentiation of adjacent cells. It has also been suggested that these cells are biochemically deficient since they have reduced levels of oxidative enzymes. This deficiency is thought to trigger a compensatory-mechanism at the organelle level in the form of mitochondrial hyperplasia. Theoretically oncocytomas could originate from oncocytes anywhere along the salivary unit or from the mature ductal cell that they most closely mimic, the striated duct cell. Against the latter is the fact that oncocytoma cells do not exhibit any other feature of the striated duct cell such as extensive basal infoldings. On the other hand cells from oncocytomas are nearly identical morphologically to oncocytes in normal glands. Also oncocytomas, like oncocytes, occur in older patients. The ultimate cell of origin for this tumor could be either the excretory duct reserve cell or the intercalated duct reserve cell. The latter cell is more since it gives rise to the salivary gland tissue where most oncocytes have been described.

Acinous cell carcinoma

Ultrastructurally, these cells contain secretory granules similar to those seen in serous acinar cells and intercalated duct cells. Secretory granules are found nowhere else in the salivary glands and hence it can be considered that the acinar cell or intercalated duct cell is the cell of origin of these neoplasms.

Adenocarcinoma

Adenocarcinomas would be expected to arise from the intercalated duct reserve cell. These neoplasms resemble more closely the undifferentiated intercalated duct cells.

References

1. Batsakis JG. Tumors of the head and neck – Clinical and pathological considerations. Williams and Wilkins, Baltimore. 1979;2(1).
2. Shafer W, Hine M, Levy B. Tumors of the salivary glands. A Textbook of Oral Pathology. Harcourt Asia Pte. Ltd. 2000;4(3)230-57.
3. Eberle RC. Parotid tumors. George GA, Editor. Current Therapy in Otolaryngology–Head and Neck Surgery, 5.pp.232-8.

Surgical pathology of salivary gland neoplasms

chapter 11

Neoplasms that arise in the salivary glands are relatively rare, yet they represent a wide variety of both benign and malignant histologic subtypes although researchers have learned much from the study of this diverse group of tumors over the years, the diagnosis and treatment of salivary gland neoplasms remain complex and challenging problems for the head and neck surgeon.

Salivary gland neoplasms make up 1% of all head and neck tumors. The incidence of salivary gland neoplasms as a whole is approximately 1.5 cases per 100,000 individuals in the United States. An estimated 700 deaths (0.4 per 100,000 for males and 0.2 per 100,000 for females) related to salivary gland tumors occur annually.

Salivary gland neoplasms most commonly appear in the sixth decade of life. Patients with malignant lesions typically present after age 60 years, whereas those with benign lesions usually present when older than 40 years. Benign neoplasms occur more frequently in woman than in men, but malignant tumors are distributed equally between the sexes.

The salivary glands are divided into 2 groups. The major salivary glands and the minor salivary glands. The major salivary glands consist of the following 3 pairs of glands. The minor salivary glands comprise 600-1000 small glands distributed throughout the upper aerodigestive tract.

Among salivary gland neoplasms, 80% arise in the parotid glands, 10-15% arises in the submandibular glands, and the remainder arises in sublingual and minor salivary glands.

Most series report that about 80% of parotid neoplasms are benign, with the relative proportion of malignance increasing in the smaller glands. A useful rule of thumb is the 25/50/75 rule. That is, as size of the gland decreases, the incidence of malignancy of a tumor in the gland increases in approximately these proportions. The most common tumor of the parotid gland is the pleomorphic adenoma. This represents about 60% of all parotid neoplasms. Almost half of all submandibular gland neoplasms and most sublingual and minor salivary gland tumors are malignant.

Salivary gland neoplasms are rare in children. Most tumors (65%) are benign, with hemangiomas being the most common, following by pleomorphic adenomas. In children, 35% of salivary gland neoplasms are malignant. Mucoepidermod carcinoma is the most common salivary gland malignancy in children.

Surgical pathology of salivary gland neoplasms

The salivary glands are the location for malignant metastases from lesions above and below the clavicle. The surgeon must have knowledge of the pathological behaviors of each tumor type in order to develop a management plan.

Successful diagnosis and treatment of patients with salivary gland tumors require a thorough understanding of tumor etiology, biologic behavior of each tumor type and salivary gland anatomy.

Normal salivary glands are made up of several different types of cells, tumors can start from any of the cell types. Salivary gland tumors are named according to which of these cell types they most look like when viewed under a microscope. The cancers are also given a numeric grade of 1, 2, 3 based on their appearance under a microscope.

- Grade 1 cancers (also called low grade or well differentiated) look very much like normal salivary gland cells and tend to grow slowly and have a good outcome.
- Grade 2 cancers (also called intermediate grade or moderately differentiated) have an appearance and outlook that is between grade 1 and grade 3 cancers.
- Grade 3 cancers (also called high grade or poorly differentiated) look quite different from normal cells, often grow and/or spread quickly, and have a poor prognosis or outlook.

The first clinical staging system was developed by Spiro and coworkers at the Memorial Hospital. The TN (Tumor, Nodes) system and TNM modification (Tumor, Nodes, Metastases) was developed for the parotid gland and submandibular glands. Consideration was given to the size of the tumor, to its mobility and to whether or not the facial nerve was intact. N_0 and N_1 designations were applied to the absence or presence of suspected cervical lymph node metastases. These criteria were accepted by American Joint Committee on Cancer in 1988. This staging system used four variables: tumor size, local extension of the tumor, the palpability of and suspected metastasis to regional lymph nodes and presence or absence of distant metastasis.[1]

In 2002, the American Joint Commission on Cancer updated the staging system for cancer of the major salivary glands. The staging system follows the tumor, node, metastasis (TNM) system of staging like other parts of the body. Primary tumor stage depends primarily on the size of the primary tumor, extraparenchymal extension and involvement of the seventh cranial nerve or skull base. Minor salivary gland tumors are staged according to the system used to classify primary tumors of those particular sites of origin, e.g. oral cavity, oropharynx, etc.[2,3]

Primary tumor (T)

TX   Primary tumor cannot be assessed
T0   No evidence of primary tumor

T1 Tumor 2 cm or less in greatest dimension without extraparenchymal extension
T2 Tumor more than 2 cm but not more than 4 cm in greatest dimension without extraparenchymal extension
T3 Tumor more than 4 cm and/or tumor having extraparenchymal extension
T4a Tumor invades skin, mandible, ear canal, and/or facial nerve
T4b Tumor invades skull base and/or pterygoid plates and/or encases carotid artery

(Extraparenchymal extension is clinical or macroscopic evidence of invasion of soft tissues or nerve, except those listed under T4a and T4b. Microscopic evidence alone does not constitute extraparenchymal extension for classification purposes).

Regional lymph nodes (N)

NX Regional lymph nodes cannot be assessed
N0 No regional lymph node metastasis
N1 Metastasis in single ipsilateral lymph node, 3 cm or less in greatest dimension
N2 Metastasis in single ipsilateral lymph node, more than 3 cm but not more than 6 cm in greatest dimension; or in multiple ipsilateral lymph nodes, none more than 6 cm in greatest dimension; or in bilateral or contralateral lymph nodes, none more than 6 cm in greatest dimension
N2a Metastasis in single ipsilateral lymph node, more than 3 cm but not more than 6 cm in greatest dimension
N2b Metastasis in multiple ipsilateral lymph nodes, none more than 6 cm in greatest dimension
N2c Metastasis in bilateral or contra lateral lymph nodes, none more than 6 cm in greatest dimension.
N3 Metastasis in a lymph node more than 6 cm in greatest dimension

(Regional nodes are the cervical nodes. Midline nodes are considered ipsilateral nodes).

Distant metastasis (M)

MX Presence of distant metastasis cannot be assessed
M0 No distant metastasis
M1 Distant metastasis

Stage grouping

Stage 1:	T1	N0	M0
Stage 2:	T2	N0	M0

Stage 3:	T3	N0	M0
	T1	N1	M0
	T2	N1	M0
	T3	N1	M0
Stage 4 A:	T4a	N0	M0
	T4a	N1	M0
	T1	N2	M0
	T2	N2	M0
	T3	N2	M0
	T4a	N2	M0
Stage 4 B:	T4b	Any N	M0
	Any T	N3	M0
Stage 4 C:	Any T	Any N	M1

Surgical pathology

A variety of benign and malignant neoplasm can arise in the salivary gland. An accurate histopathology diagnosis is essential for the rational treatment of patients with salivary gland neoplasm. Batsakis et al have reported the classification system most commonly used in epithelial salivary gland tumors.

Pleomorphic adenoma

The pleomorphic tumor or benign mixed tumor is the most common tumor of salivary gland origin. It represents over half of the parotid tumors.[4] Approximately 65 percent patients of salivary gland neoplasms are classified as benign mixed tumors or pleomorphic adenoma.[5] The tumor derives its name from the Greek words Pleos = many and morphus = form because of the heterogeneous nature of its histologic appearance.[6] The term "Pleomorphic Adenoma" suggested by Willis closely resembles the unusual Histologic pattern of the lesion.[7] The term Benign mixed tumor was proposed by Broca in 1866 and Minssen in 1874 to describe the two components of the tumor, mesenchymal and epithelial.[8,9]

Definition

Tumor of variable capsulation characterized microscopically by architectural rather than cellular pleomorphism. Epithelial and myoepithelial elements intermingle most commonly with tissue of mucoid, myxoid or chondroid appearance.

Clinical features

It presents as a firm, slowly growing mass that frequently has been present asymptomatically for few years. They are most frequently found in the parotid gland, then the submandibular gland followed by the minor salivary glands. They also represent the most common tumor of each gland composing 77 percent of parotid gland tumors, 60 percent of submandibular gland tumors and 53 percent of tumors arising in the palate.[9] In a case series of 4245 cases of pleomorphic adenoma reported by Nauch 92.5% of cases were seen in major salivary glands and 6.5% of cases are seen in minor glands. 84% were reported in the parotid gland, 8% in the submandibular gland and 0.5% in the sublingual gland.[5] Incidence of the tumor except those found in the pharynx is more in females than males and they are often seen in the fourth and fifth decade. A bilateral tumor occurrence rate is estimated at 1 in 40,000.[8,10]

In the parotid gland, the lesion most commonly involves the superficial portion of the gland lateral to the facial nerve. The pleomorphic adenoma is slow growing tumor which is intermittent in growth or the growth may even seem to be phasic.[8,10] On gross inspection they are smooth, rounded and lobular and mobile with a rubbery consistency. The surface may be smooth or multilobulated **(Figures 11. 1 and 11.2)**. If the tumor involves both, the superficial as well as deep lobe of parotid, it is classically referred to as dumbbell tumor **(Figure 11.3)**.

They are encapsulated but often have some pseudopod formations at the periphery that can lead to a less than complete removal and subsequent recurrence.[4] The tumor does not show fixity to the deeper tissues or the overlying skin. However in tumors of the minor salivary glands of the palate, it may appear to be fixed to the underlying palatal bone but does not

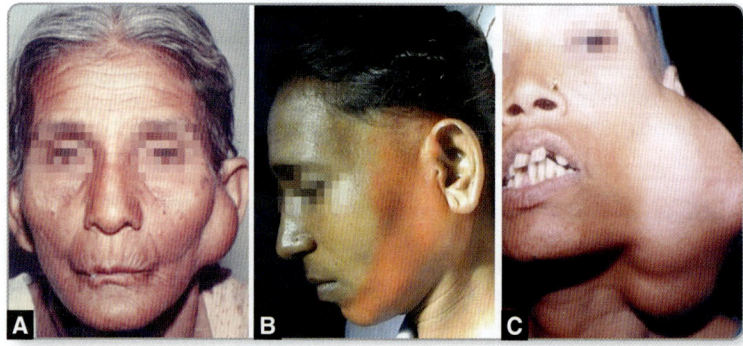

Figures 11.1A to C Various presentations of pleomorphic adenoma of parotid gland (A, B) Smooth surface; (C) Multilobulated surface (*Courtesy:* Dr. Suhas Jajoo)

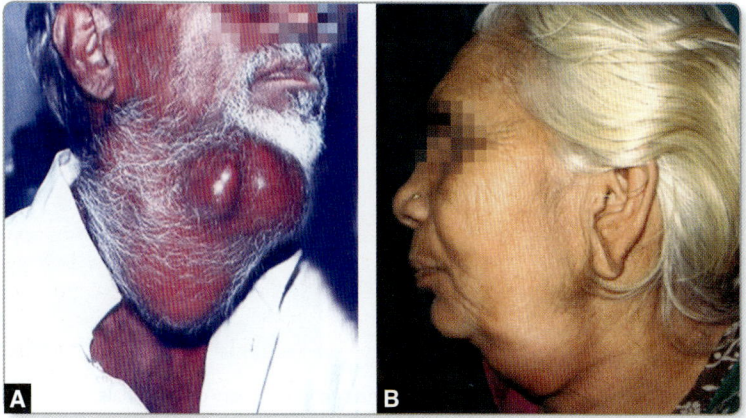

Figures 11.2A and B Pleomorphic adenoma of submandibular gland (A) Multilobulated surface; (B) Smooth surface

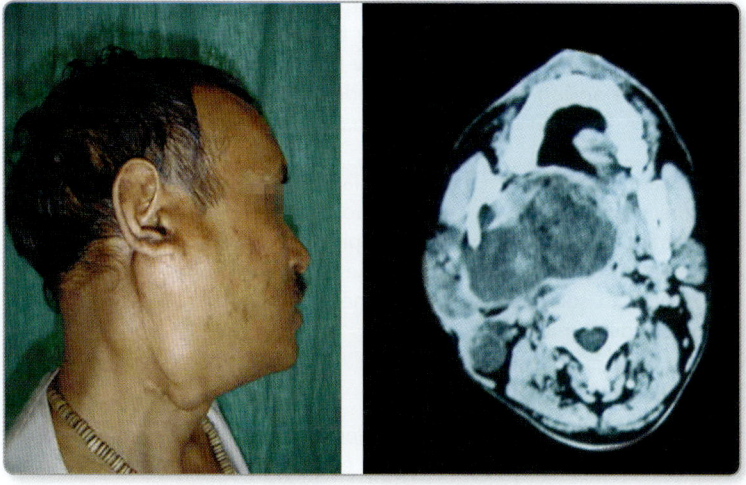

Figure 11.3 Dumb-bell tumor of parotid gland

invade or erode the bone **(Figure 11.4)**. Pain is not a common feature but approximately 50 percent of the patients experience a pressure sensation. The lesion may be sensitive when palpated. Accumulation of mucus can occur so that elastic swellings or frankly fluctuant cysts may form in the tumors. Chen and Loucks, in 1933, stated that mixed tumors may vary from the size of an olive to the size of an adult person's head.[11] The overlying skin

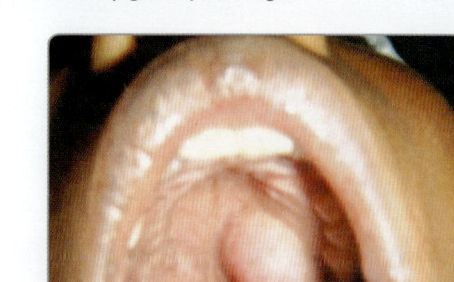
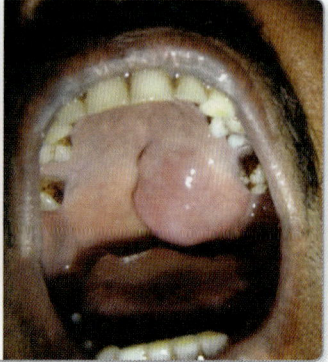

Figure 11.4 Pleomorphic adenoma of minor salivary gland of palate
(*Courtesy:* Dr. Suhas Jajoo)

seldom ulcerates even though the tumor might assume a massive size.[7] Benign lymphadenopathy is seen due to reactive hyperplasia associated with stasis produced by duct obstruction.[11] According to Thackray and Sabin, 1972, after around 20–30 years a few tumors may suddenly and rapidly increase in size, accompanied by new invasive growth. This is described as carcinoma arising in pleomorphic adenoma. Majority of tumors do not metastasize, however multiple pulmonary metastases may be seen which are fatal.[10]

In case of the submandibular gland, palpation of the mass both extraorally and bimanually helps in localizing it. At times it is difficult to differentiate it from enlarged lymph nodes overlying the gland and inflammatory disease of the gland if the patient has no history of recurrent sialadenitis. In such cases FNAC of the gland can be used to solve the diagnostic dilemma.

Gross pathology[12]

Surgically excised pleomorphic adenomas usually range from 2–5 cm in diameter. They are ovoid, smooth, encapsulated, multi-lobulated. The capsule is thin and delicate, but can be focally thick. Small excrescences are seen jutting out from the external surface of the capsule.

Cut section of the tumor shows a moist and gray white surface with a faint yellow cast **(Figure 11.5)**. When cartilage like material is present the surface is translucent with a bluish hue. Cyst formation and hemorrhage are infrequent but do occur in large tumors. In tumors with a prominent myxoid or mucinous stroma the cut surface appears slimy. Occasionally tumors are firm and resemble myxomas or fibrous lesions. Primary tumors are usually single. In contrast recurrences are frequently multiple tumor masses.

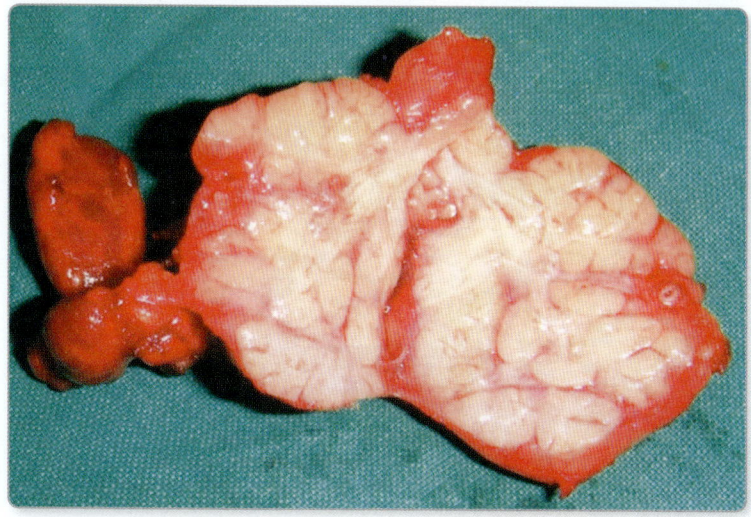

Figure 11.5 Cut section of pleomorphic adenoma
(*Courtesy:* Dr. Suhas Jajoo)

Histopathology[12]

The diverse histologic pattern is the most characteristic feature of this tumor **(Figure 11.6)**. Rarely do two individual tumors resemble each other.[8] On light microscopy morphologically complex and diverse cellular elements are seen. Both epithelial and myoepithelial elements are present. Their relative proportions vary widely. Based on cellular types Foote and Frazel have classified pleomorphic adenomas as follows:
1. Principally myxoid (36%)
2. Equally myxoid and cellular (30%)
3. Predominantly cellular (20%)
4. Extremely cellular (12%)
5. Predominantly composed of elongated spindle shaped cells growing in anastomosing bands and bundles (1%) – first described by Bauer and Fox.

Two types of cells compose a majority of pleomorphic adenomas, an inner row of epithelial cells and an outer layer of myoepithelial cells. Some areas present cuboidal cells arranged in tubes or duct like structures that bear striking resemblance to the normal ductal epithelium. These duct like spaces not uncommonly contain an eosinophilic coagulum. There is often proliferation of epithelium in strands or sheets about these tubular structures. In other areas the tumor cells assume a stellate, polyhedral

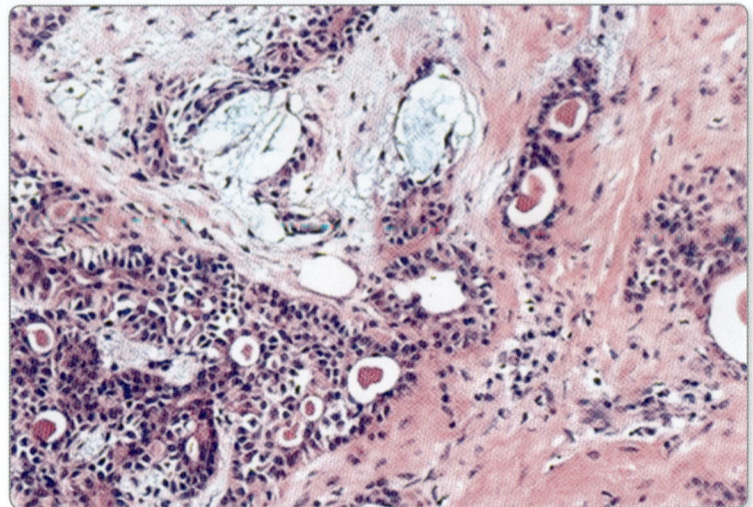

Figure 11.6 Photomicrograph of pleomorphic adenoma (40X)
(*Source:* Ellis GL, Editor. Surgical pathology of the salivary glands)

or spindle form and may be relatively few in number. A hyaline cell with plasmacytoid morphology has also been described in 70% and 10% of minor and major pleomorphic adenomas respectively by Lomax-Smith and Azzopardi. On ultrastructural analysis Buchner et al suggested that the hyaline cells are modified myoepithelial cells. Squamous epithelial cells are seen which exhibit intercellular bridges and sometimes actual keratin pearls. Loose myxoid material is predominantly seen in these tumors and foci of hyalinized connective tissue or cartilage or osseous components may also be seen. In addition, a mucoid material secreted by cells can get accumulated in areas. The tumor is always encapsulated, the fibrous capsule being of variable thickness, completeness and density; however, tumor cells are often present in the capsular connective tissue. Compression of surrounding tissue and focal capsular defects produce an impression of invasion.

Immunoprofile[13]

Inner ductal cells in the tubulo glandular structures are positive for cytokeratin 3, 6, 10, 11, 13 and 16, whereas the neoplastic myoepithelial cells are irregularly positive for cytokeratin 13, 16 and 14. Neoplastic myoepithelial cells co expressvimentin and pancytokeratin.

Molecular genetics[13]
Target gene in pleomorphic adenomas with 8q 12 is P2AG1.

Management of pleomorphic adenoma of parotid gland
The treatment of choice for pleomorphic adenomas primarily is surgery. Until 1930 the method of choice of treating pleomorphic adenomas of the parotid gland was enucleation. In 1936, McFarland put light on the high incidence of recurrences associated with enucleation. Patey and Thackray, in 1957, explained this by demonstrating a lack of capsular integrity and microscopic tumor extensions beyond the main body of the mass. Thus surgery close to the tumor mass was considered inadequate with risk of rupture, tumor dissemination and a high risk of recurrence.[14]

Since most recurrences are traced to enucleation of the tumor, it is excised along with a thick collar of normal tissue. Majority of pleomorphic adenomas in the parotid gland occur in the superficial portion of the gland lateral to the facial nerve.[8] In such cases resection of the tumor is carried out of the entire superficial portion lateral to the facial nerve.

Superficial parotidectomy is the most widely accepted technique in the treatment of pleomorphic adenomas in the superficial lobe of the parotid gland. Other techniques are enucleation, pericapsular excision, total parotidectomy with facial nerve preservation and partial superficial parotidectomy.[14]

In a study by Matsuura H from 1970–1983 the surgical treatments for the pleomorphic adenomas were 11 extirpations and 45 parotidectomies. The recurrence in each treatment was observed in one (9%) and in none (0%), respectively. The average follow-up period is 11 years (from 5 to 19). The treatment of choice for pleomorphic adenoma is parotidectomy of the superficial, deep and/or posterior lobes.[12]

In literature opinion is divided, whether for treatment of pleomorphic adenoma in the parotid gland partial parotidectomy is adequate or complete parotidectomy is necessary. In a retrospective analysis of 123 complete parotidectomies in pleomorphic adenomas the macroscopic tumor extension was compared with the microscopic findings. Additionally 35 pleomorphic adenomas were examined in histological serial sections. The retrospective analysis showed in 6%, the serial sections in 11% microscopic tumor in the macroscopic tumor free inner lobe in a clinical follow-up examination of 85 patients operated by complete parotidectomy because pleomorphic adenoma resulted in a relapse-quota of 3.5%. The function of the facial nerve was in most cases normal; in 8.2% a weakness of the mandibular branch was found. These results indicate that the risk to leave tumor can be reduced evidently by a complete parotidectomy.[15]

Management of pleomorphic adenoma of submandibular gland

Tumors of the submandibular gland are usually contained within the gland and their resection is usually confined to the gland and surrounding fat or lymph nodes until the neoplasm is a malignant and invasive tumor. As with the parotid gland most neoplasms are asymptomatic.

Management of pleomorphic adenomas of the palate

Small palatal pleomorphic adenomas usually cause pressure resorption of the palate but do not invade the bone. A disc of palatal mucosa is outlined well clear of the visible swelling because the tumor is flattened owing to the toughness of the palatal tissues. The tumor along with the periosteum of the palate is excised in continuity with each other. In case the pleomorphic adenoma invades the palate or proliferates into the floor of the maxillary sinus, a partial maxillectomy or total maxillectomy depending on the extension of the tumor has to be performed.

Prognosis

Although pleomorphic adenoma is a benign tumor, it may cause problems in clinical management due to its tendency to recur and risk of malignant transformation. **Figures 11.7A and B** shows a recurrent pleomorphic adenoma in a child of 10 years age.

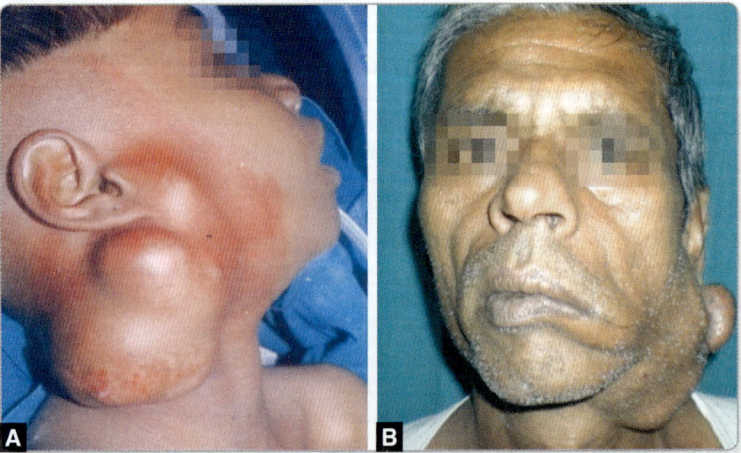

Figures 11.7A and B (A) Recurrent pleomorphic adenoma in a child (Note scar from previous surgery) (*Courtesy:* Dr Suhas Jajoo); (B) Recurrent malignant pleomorphic adenoma

Warthin's tumor

Warthin's tumor, also known as papillary cystadenoma lymphomatosum is the second most common benign tumor of the salivary glands.[16] This tumor was first described by Hildebrand in 1895 as a form of congenital cyst of the neck. In 1910 Albrecht and Arzt described two cases as papillary cystadenoma of lymphoid stroma and considered the lesions to be of pharyngeal endodermal anlagen. The first cases reported in English language literature were reported by Nicholson in 1923 as adenomas of heterotopic salivary glands.[17] However in America it is known as Warthin's tumor in recognition of the pathologist who first described it in the US in 1929.[18] He described two cases and also coined the term papillary cystadenoma lymphomatosum.[17] They constitute only 5% of the salivary gland neoplasms.[19] The British term adenolymphoma has been adopted in the WHO and AFIP classification but suffers the disadvantage of utilizing a verbal form with confusing malignant connotations for a benign tumor. Chaudhary and Gorlin reviewed the world literature in 1958 and cited 23 synonyms for this neoplasm. Most frequently used synonyms are cystic papillary adenoma, papillary cystadenoma lymphomatosum, branchial cysts of the parotid, branchiogenic adenoma, onkocytoma, adenolymphoma, lymphoglandular cystome and Warthin's tumor. Papillary cystadenoma lymphomatosum is now the most appropriate term because it is fully descriptive of the tumor.[17] This tumor is one of the most readily identifiable tumors of the salivary gland.

Clinical features

The majority of the tumors arise in the parotid gland, the incidence being 2 to 15 percent of all parotid gland tumors. Warthin described only 2 cases out of 700 whereas Orloff reported an incidence of 2–6 percent of parotid tumors and 1.6–4.2 percent of all salivary gland tumors. Most of the studies have shown an occurrence rate of 5 to 6 percent in the parotid gland. John Saunders et al have reported papillary cystadenoma lymphomatosum or Warthin's tumor to be found only in the parotid gland although cases have been reported in submandibular gland too.[20,21]

It has long been considered to be a tumor of the elderly and occurs rarely before the third decade. Most tumors are reported in the fifth and sixth decades of life. A predilection for male sex is seen, the ratio being reported as high as 10:1 to 5:1 in older literature. Recently this has changed to 1.5:1.[22] Racial statistics indicates that Warthin's tumor occurs predominantly amongst whites. It does occur bilaterally with a frequency of 5–14 percent. However both the tumors do not occur simultaneously, but are metachronous in their manifestation. A concept of multicentric and multifocal disease has been put forth to explain the bilateral occurrence of the tumor.

Similar to any other parotid tumor, papillary cystadenoma lymphomatosum is a solitary, nodular, slowly enlarging swelling. A typical Warthin's tumor in the parotid gland is located in the inferior pole of the parotid next to the angle of the mandible and is usually 2–3 cm in size at the time of diagnosis. It varies from moderately firm to fluctuant on palpation and is asymptomatic. It is not as discrete as the mixed tumor. Very few patients, less than 10%, present with complain of pain, pressure or rapid increase in the tumor size. In cases of the tumor being located inferior to and outside the parotid gland, the clinical diagnosis may be more in favor of branchial cleft cyst, chronic lymphadenitis, lymphoma or tuberculosis.

Sialography is not useful in distinguishing the tumor from other salivary gland tumors. However scintigraphy may be helpful in differentiating adenolymphoma lymphomatosum due to its increased uptake of technetium-99m pertechnetate. It appears as a smooth-margined, radiopositive "hot" nodule in contrast to the mixed tumors, non functioning malignant tumors and metastatic tumors which appears as a "cold" nodule in scintigraphy. Positive scintigraphy with ^{123}I is indicative of Warthin's tumor but may also signify presence of ectopic thyroid or metastatic thyroid tumor.

Gross pathology[17]

The surgical specimen is usually a spherical or oval mass that is covered by a thin, tough capsule, which is usually intact. The tumor has a smooth, red gray, lobulated surface. Tumor consistency varies from fluctuant in specimens with a single large cystic space to firm and rubbery in more solid tumors with small or few cysts. The cut surface of the tumor is pathognomonic and varies with the presence of small cysts varying in number and size. Cut surface also

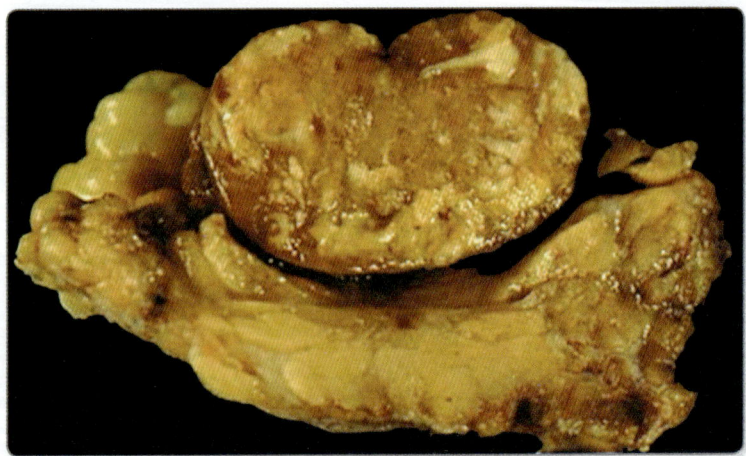

Figure 11.8 Cut section of Warthin's tumor

shows papillary projections. Rarely a single cyst is present. However, usually multiple small cysts are present which vary in size from few millimeter to a centimeter in diameter. The cystic compartment contains fluid of variable viscosity that may be clear, serous, mucoid, brown-tinged (chocolate) or semisolid caseous material. The linings of the cyst appear shaggy and irregular with multiple intricate papillae that extend from the cyst wall. The solid portions of the tumor are gray-white and correspond to the lymphoid component. Within the solid areas, these nodules represent lymphoid follicles. Papillary cystadenoma lymphomatosum can be diagnosed grossly unless liquefaction is present which may give the impression of tuberculous lymphadenitis or branchial cleft cyst.

Histopathology[17]

Warthin's tumor is made of two histologic components viz: epithelial and lymphoid. As the name suggests, it is an adenoma which exhibits cyst formation with papillary projections into the cystic spaces and a lymphoid matrix with germinal centers. The epithelial cells covering the papillary projections are tall columnar or cuboidal cells arranged in two rows. Tall columnar cells approximate the cystic spaces. They are eosinophilic containing hyperchromatic or pkynotic nuclei that are placed near the luminal space and vast number of mitochondria as seen under electron microscope. The inner cells are cuboidal and polygonal and contain nuclei

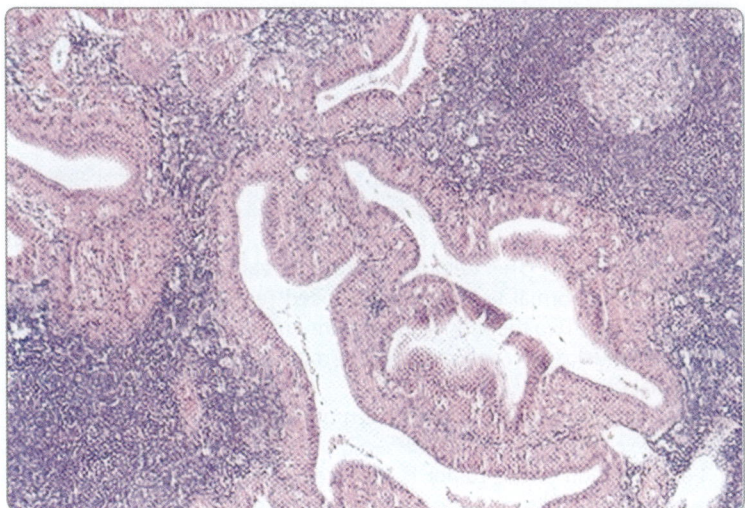

Figure 11.9 Photomicrograph of Warthin's tumor (40X)
(*Source:* Ellis GL, Editor. Surgical pathology of the salivary glands)

with prominent nucleoli. Both cell layers have finely granular and distinctly eosinophilic cytoplasm. Frequently, an eosinophilic coagulum is present within the cystic spaces which appear as a chocolate colored fluid in the gross specimen and is PAS (per acid-Schiff) stain positive. Luminal cells are rarely ciliated but show a fuzzy luminal surface which is attributed to presence of microvilli. The abundant lymphoid component may represent normal lymphoid tissue of the lymph node within which the tumor developed or it may actually represent a reactive cellular infiltrate which involves both humoral and cell mediated mechanisms. It is separated from the cellular component by a thin basement membrane.

The most frequent histologic variations in papillary cystadenoma lymphomatosum are oncocytosis, squamous metaplasia, mucous cell prosoplasia and rarely inclusions of sebaceous glands. Oncocytosis is characterized by sheets and nests of disorganized oncocytic cells that show loss of papillary formation. Focal oncocytosis within the tumor should not be construed as a separate neoplasm or as a malignant degeneration. This tumor frequently shows focal areas of squamous metaplasia, presenting as a flattened, and luminal surface with loss of regimented columnar cells. When associated with inflammation it may show squamous metaplasia and spontaneous necrosis. In areas of metaplasia the squamous cells have uniformly bland cytologic features. If cellular atypia is encountered, possibility of malignant transformation should be considered. However, a diagnosis of malignancy depends on the presence of stromal invasion or metastasis. Malignant tumors arising in these tumors are squamous cell carcinoma, undifferentiated carcinoma, adenocarcinoma and mucoepidermoid carcinoma. Histochemical studies are of little significance in diagnosis of Warthin's tumor.

Management of Warthin's tumor

The established treatment for Warthin's tumor is surgical removal. Because most tumors are located superficially in the parotid gland the tumor is easily removed with minimal loss of glandular function and with preservation of the facial nerve. The debate regarding treatment usually concerns the amount of normal tissue to be removed required to attain minimal recurrence rates. Two theories of surgical treatment are: [23]
1. Tumor enucleation with resection of minimal amount of surrounding normal tissue.
2. Superficial parotidectomy, which is more aggressive than enucleation.
3. Local excision of parotid gland[23]

Local excision of the tumor is preferred to enucleation of the tumor because lymph nodes at the posteroinferior part of the gland cannot be cleared by enucleation.[23]

Preoperatively diagnosis of Warthin's tumor must be confirmed by coordinating the clinical findings with imaging and fine needle aspiration biopsy reports before local excision is carried out. Few patients of Warthin's tumor have associated chronic obstructive parotitis. If the sialogram shows obvious irregular dilation of the main duct then superficial parotidectomy is essential. Similarly, if the tumor is located in front of the ear, a superficial parotidectomy is the treatment of choice.

Oncocytoma

An oncocytoma is a tumor characterized by large epithelial cells i.e. oncocytes that contain a brightly eosinophilic, granular cytoplasm. The oncocyte which is derived from the Greek word "onkousthai" meaning swollen or enlarged was initially described in 1897 by Schaffer who observed this tumor in ductal and acinar elements of salivary glands in the tongue, pharynx and esophagus. This histopathology of this tumor was also noted by Zimmermann, who noticed the presence of cells with condensed nuclear chromatin or pyknotic nuclei and hence termed them 'pkynocytes'. Jaffe was the first to introduce the term oncocytoma. However, he had termed Warthin's tumor as oncocytoma. The first case report of oncocytoma was described by McFarland in 1927, but this terminology was not used.[24]

In 1931, Hamperl first applied the term 'onkocyte' to cells which make up the oncocytoma. He noted these cells in salivary glands of individuals in the sixth decade as well as in the tissues such as kidneys, thyroid, parathyroid, pituitary and adrenal glands and tumors affecting these glands.

The other terminologies used to describe this tumor are oxyphilic adenoma, acidophilic adenoma.[25]

Clinical features

There have been numerous studies which indicate that this tumor occurs uncommonly. Evidence from data gathered from large series indicates that this tumor is predominantly observed in the elderly population with distribution over sixth, seventh and eight decades of life. At AFIP the age distribution of oncocytoma has been observed to be from sixth to ninth decades, the highest percentage (31.3%) of cases being found in the ninth decade. Oncocytomas make up 2.3% of benign epithelial tumors and are among the least common types of benign salivary gland tumors.[24]

There is no race predilection for occurrence of this tumor. It occurs predominantly in females as reported by Evans and Cruickshank as also by Eneroth, Hamperl and Chaudhry and Gorlin. However, Lane's evaluation suggests an equal distribution in males and females.

Oncocytoma is predominantly a tumor of the major salivary glands. Most of the tumors are found in the parotid gland, but they have also been reported in the submandibular gland. Studies have reported a bilateral occurrence of oncocytoma in the parotid gland.[26] Amongst minor salivary glands, which are rarely affected, palatal mucosa is the most common location followed by buccal mucosa and tongue.

The oncocytoma is a small benign lesion which generally does not attain a great size. It is clinically indistinguishable from other benign neoplasms of the major salivary glands. It most frequently presents as an indolent, single, often multilobulated, firm, solid mass in the superficial lobe of the parotid gland. It can also be located in the deep lobe of the parotid gland and may be insinuated between the branches of the facial nerve. However it does not cause any symptoms of pain or paresthesia unless the branches of the facial nerve are compromised. Tumor size varies with the duration of the lesion but generally does not increase beyond 4.0 cm. It is usually freely movable on palpation. A condition called "oncocytosis" or "diffuse multinodular oncocytoma" of the parotid gland has been described by Schwartz and Feldman wherein nodules of oncocytes involve the entire gland or large portions of it.[25]

Intraoral tumors do not exhibit any special characteristic diagnostic features. However their overlying mucosa may become ulcerated due to trauma.[24]

Grove and Di Chiro as also other research workers have shown that oncocytoma and Warthin's tumor show an increased uptake of pertechnetate anion from the technetium-99m pertechnetate scintigraphy and show evidence of hot spot. However, it has also been shown that hot spots are seen in case of malignant tumors also.

Gross pathology[24]

External surface of the tumor is smooth and may be multinodular and lobulated. The cut surface is white-gray with focal areas of red-brown hemorrhage. It is generally homogenous in consistency and demonstrates distinct intersecting fibrous connective tissue septa within the tumor mass. A tumor in the minor salivary gland is usually solid but may also show a cystic component. It is covered by oral mucosa unless secondarily ulcerated. The tumor is well defined but might not be completely encapsulated. In case of palatal tumor pressure resorption of the bone might be evident but there is no invasion of bone.

Histopathology[24]

It is a well circumscribed tumor that is composed of oncocytes arranged in solid sheets or in nests and cords which form alveolar or organoid patterns. Some of these structures may have small central lumina. A mild, chronic inflammatory cell infiltrate may be present. The oncocyte is a large, well defined, polyhedral or round cell that is characterized by brightly eosinophilic cytoplasm with prominent granularity. The intensity of cytoplasmic granularity is proportional to degree of cytoplasmic granularity. Individual oncocytes appear adherent closely and have distinct cellular boundaries unless the tissue has been poorly preserved wherein acantholysis may be noted. Cells with clear cytoplasm are scattered focally throughout the tumor or may be seen as solid masses.

Groups of oncocytes are supported by numerous, thin, fibrous connective tissue septa that contain small endothelium-lined vascular spaces. A centrally located nucleus may be small and hyperchromatic or large and vesiculated with prominent nucleoli. Few mitoses are observed. Some degree of increased cellular atypia, nuclear hyperchromatism and pleomorphism is accepted as compatible with benignancy in oncocytoma. In absence of infiltration these atypical histopathologic features are not suggestive of malignancy. The cytoplasmic granularity is due to packing of the cytoplasm with mitochondria which occupy up to 60 percent of the total cell volume.

Azzopardi and Smith have demonstrated that oncocytoma gives a positive reaction for glycogen if stained by periodic acid-schiff reagent before and after digestion with diastase. Staining for acid mucopolysaccharides with alcian blue and mucicarmine stains produce a negative result.

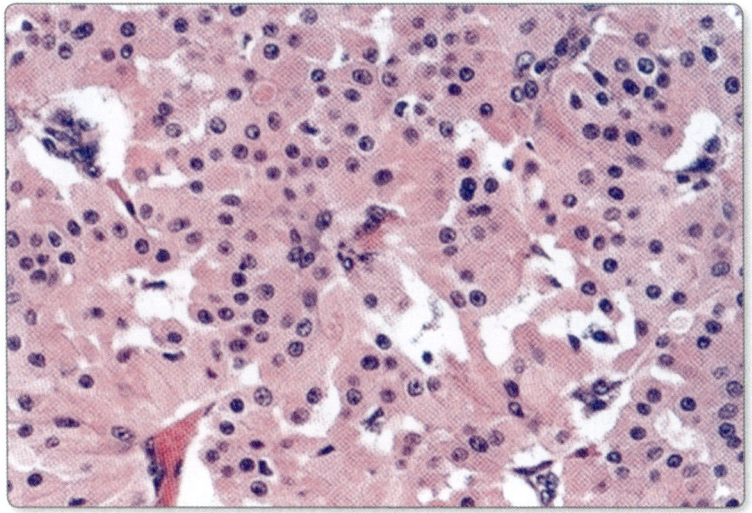

Figure 11.10 Photomicrograph of oncocytoma (40X)
(*Source:* Ellis GL, Editor. Surgical pathology of the salivary glands)

Management of oncocytoma

Surgery is the most common and accepted treatment for oncocytoma. Although most parotid oncocytomas are encapsulated and located superficially, partial parotidectomy with facial nerve preservation whenever possible is the treatment of choice. It ensures complete removal of the tumor and reduces the rate of recurrence. Curettage or simple enucleation of the tumor is to be avoided to avoid recurrence. If the facial nerve is to be sacrificed, microneurosurgical repair is considered. Complete glandectomy is the treatment of choice in cases of submandibular gland oncocytomas. In case of minor gland tumors, local excision of the tumor with a margin of normal tumor-free tissue is carried out. Radiation therapy after surgery has been tried but it has been shown to be ineffective.

Monomorphic adenoma

The term monomorphic adenoma was first suggested by Thackray and Sobin in the World Health Organization monograph on salivary gland tumors. The WHO classification subdivides the monomorphic adenomas into three groups:[27]
1. Adenolymphoma (Warthin's tumor)
2. Oxyphilic adenoma (Oncocytoma)
3. Others.

The first two are separate well recognized entities. A number of other classifications of monomorphic adenomas have been put forth, but there is no unanimity. Two main histologic patterns have evolved:
a. Basal cell adenoma
b. Canalicular adenoma.

Basal cell adenoma

It was first reported as a separate entity by Kleinsasser and Klein in 1967. Batsakis has described the first case in American literature, wherein he has suggested that the intercalated duct or reserve cell is the histogenetic source of the tumor.[27]

Clinical features

They constitute approximately 1.8% of all benign primary epithelial salivary gland tumors in the AFIP records. Other studies have shown that its incidence is between 1.8 and 7.5 percent of all salivary gland tumors. Basal cell adenomas have a propensity to occur in major salivary gland tumors, more so in the parotid gland like most other tumors. As per the AFIP registry 73.1 percent of the basal cell adenomas occur in the parotid gland.[28] In a series of basal cell adenomas reported by Batsakis and associates, 48 out of 50 tumors were located in the parotid gland and the other two in the submandibular gland.[27] The average age of occurrence of this tumor is between third and ninth decade, but the peak incidence is seen in the sixth decade.[2] There is a male predilection of 5:1.[27] However in the AFIP registry records are suggestive of a higher predilection in females (66.2%). Daley and coworkers have reported an equal distribution in either sex whereas Luna and colleagues have suggested 90% incidence in males.[28]

Basal cell adenomas are clinically indistinguishable from mixed tumors. They tend to occur in the superficial portion of the parotid gland and are freely movable. They do not show any predisposition for occurrence on any particular side of the salivary glands. They appear as a round or ovoid, well circumscribed mass with a smooth-surfaced capsule and a soft to moderately firm consistency. Their greatest dimension is usually less than 3 cm, ranging from 1.2 cm to 8.0 cm and may be mistaken for a hyperplastic lymph node because of their encapsulation and color. They are characterized by slow growth and are usually painless.

Gross pathology[28]

The cut surface of the tumor has a homogenous, solid appearance that may show cysts of varying sizes. The cysts may be filled with brown/red mucinous material or blood. The color of the cut surface may vary from gray-white to pink-red or brown. However it tends to be uniform.

Histopathological features[28]

On the basis of their morphologic appearance they may be divided into four subtypes:
1. Solid
2. Trabecular
3. Tubular
4. Membranous.

In spite of these morphologically variable forms, basic histological features are characteristic and facilitate the diagnosis. The cells that make up the tumor are uniform and regular from tumor to tumor. These basaloid cells have morphologic forms that are intermixed. The larger, pale cells generally predominate with the smaller, darker cells often located in the peripheral portions of the epithelial tumor nests, cords or islands. Often the nuclei have a slightly irregular outline and may have a grooved appearance. One or two chromatin condensations may be seen or nuclei may have small eosinophilic nucleoli. Rarely mitosis may be seen.

There is a sharp demarcation between the neoplastic epithelial cells and the surrounding connective tissue. Also there is a palisading of peripheral cuboidal or slightly columnar cells that accentuates the epithelial-connective tissue interface.

The most common type of basal cell adenoma is a solid variant which consists of islands and cords of neoplastic epithelial cells that have a broad, rounded, lobular pattern. The hyperchromatic peripheral layers of cells which are either cuboidal or columnar often demonstrate palisading. The inner layer of epithelial cells appears to have a directional orientation that tends to parallel the basilar cells. In few tumors these cells form whorls which may mature in to squamous cells and produce keratin to give the appearance of small keratin cysts or keratin pearls.

The trabecular type of tumor has histologic features similar to the solid variety but the epithelial islands are narrower and cord like and form interconnecting tongue like islands with rounded borders. These strands of epithelium may be only two cells thick in a few areas. In areas where they are thick, the picture resembles a solid tumor.

The tubular pattern exhibits multiple small, round, duct-like structures. Sometimes this pattern may be seen together with the trabecular pattern to form a trabeculo-tubular composite.

The membranous basal cell adenomas have a microscopic picture similar to the dermal cylindroma. At low magnification, it appears similar to the solid variant with an exception that it is usually multilobular and is encapsulated in only half the cases. The epithelial islands are arranged in large lobules that appear to mold to the shape of the other lobules forming a jigsaw puzzle pattern. The cells are regular in pattern but the peripheral palisaded cells have a darker, more compact appearance whereas the central cells are slightly larger with lighter nuclei. It has a thick eosinophilic hyaline layer that surrounds the epithelial islands and separates these islands from each other. This hyaline material stains positive for PAS stain. Similar PAS positive material is seen within the epithelial islands and appears like hyaline droplets. In few cases these hyaline droplets coalesce and produce large eosinophilic masses.

Differential diagnosis

Basal cell carcinoma of skin, ameloblastoma, pleomorphic adenoma and adenoid cystic carcinoma should be ruled out.[29] The first two can be differentiated based on site of origin and histopathology. Pleomorphic adenoma is differentiated based on histopathology. ACC presents with microcysts and invasive growth on histopathological examination.

Management of basal cell adenomas

The neoplasm is treated by surgical excision with a sufficient clear margin of normal tissue. Thackray and Lucas have suggested that surgery for basal cell adenoma should be on lines of mixed tumor to avoid incomplete removal or tumor implantation in to the surrounding wound tissues which would result in to recurrence.

Canalicular adenoma

Clinical features

The average age of a patient affected by Canalicular adenoma is 65 years i.e. in the seventh decade. However it is seen between the fourth and ninth decade. There is a predilection for occurrence of the tumor in the female sex with a female: male ratio of 1.7 to 1.0. Others have reported a female to male ratio of 1.2 to 1.8. They have a higher incidence of occurrence in the white race as compared to blacks. [30]

The most common site of occurrence is upper lip, followed by the buccal mucosa as seen in a study conducted at AFIP. Occurrence of this tumor in the major salivary glands including the parotid gland is quite minimal.[31]

The canalicular adenoma presents as a non-ulcerated, painless nodule that exhibits slow growth. The lesion rarely shows ulceration or necrosis of the overlying mucosa, although traumatized lesions may exhibit surface ulceration and necrosis. The size of the lesion varies between 0.4 and 2.0 cm. Canalicular adenomas may give a clinical appearance of a mucocele.[32] The overlying mucosa may be normal colored or bluish. They are often freely movable and unattached to the underlying skin.[30]

Gross pathology[30]

Grossly it appears like a discrete encapsulated nodule. It may be noncapsulated but circumscribed. They are rarely multinodular or multimodal. The color has been reported to range from pink-tan to tan, brown or yellow. On cut section the nodule often shows cystic spaces and gelatinous mucoid material. In case of multifocal canalicular adenomas, larger foci are encapsulated while smaller foci are non capsulated and appear as the nidus of proliferation of salivary gland parenchyma. This should not be considered as a feature of malignancy.

Histopathology[30]

Microscopically the cells are isomorphic and cuboidal to columnar, with moderate to sparse eosinophilic cytoplasm that contains scattered granules that stain positive with PAS stain. These granules are diastase labile indicating them to be glycogen. The cell boundaries are usually indistinct. The basophilic nuclei are regular, ovoid and elongated. The chromatin is diffuse and lightly granular. Rarely scattered nuclei may show vesiculation.

Quite often the nuclei are aligned in two different levels giving the appearance of pseudostratified epithelium. Mitoses are rare. The epithelium is clearly demarcated from the fibrous connective tissue stroma. At a low magnification, cells appear arranged in cords or columns in a single layer. In many rows the single rows of cells are parallel, forming long 'canals' with central lumina. Hence the tumor is referred to as 'canalicular' adenoma. Multiple, small cystic spaces may give it a micro cystic appearance whereas a large cystic space may give it a cystic appearance, both on gross appearance as well as under the microscope. When cystic, the tumors may have papillary projections in to the lumina. These projections are covered by the same columnar or cuboidal cells that make up the body of the neoplasm. In these areas psammoma bodies may be seen. Occasionally mucous cells or oncocytic cells may be seen.

In some tumors more solid cellular proliferation may be present which show features of both canalicular as well as basal cell adenomas. Stroma shows sparse fibrillarity, lack of cellularity and prominent vascularity. It shows few fibroblasts and minimal to moderate collagen. Few areas may even show inflammatory changes such as edematous, lightly basophilic cells with few scattered inflammatory cells. The relatively acellular stroma stains with mucicarmine, alcain blue and PAS with or without diastase predigestion. The loose fibrous connective tissue stroma contains numerous delicate, endothelium lined vascular spaces, some of which appear engorged with blood. Hemosiderin deposits are seen in foci of macrophages or as finely granular pigment found apparently within epithelial cells. This apparent epithelial pigmentation resembles melanin, but iron stains confirm its true nature.

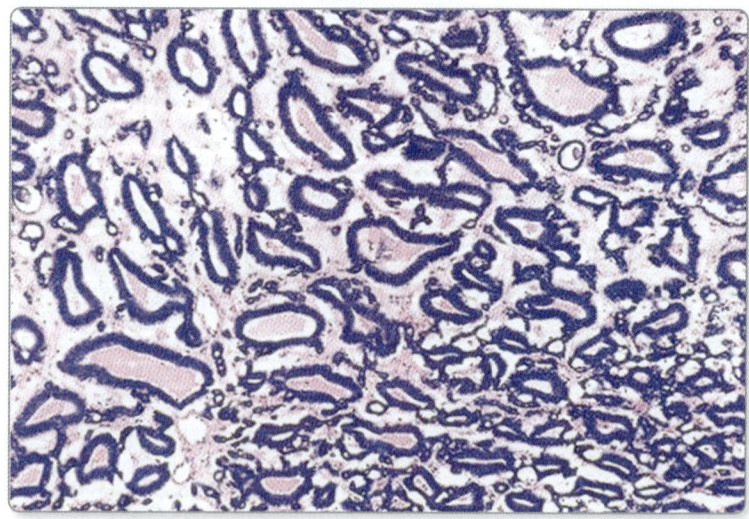

Figure 11.11 Photomicrograph of canalicular adenoma (40X)
(*Source:* Ellis GL, Editor. Surgical pathology of the salivary glands)

Differential diagnosis

In case of upper lip, a D/D of sialolith, mucocele, mucous retention cyst and pleomorphic adenoma should be considered. Sialolith of sufficient size is radiopaque whereas canalicular adenoma is radiolucent. In addition it is associated with pain and inflammation unlike the latter. Mucocele and mucous retention cysts may mimic cystic type of canalicular adenoma but are uncommon in the upper lip and occur in a younger age group. Also they are freely movable below the overlying mucosa. It can be differentiated from pleomorphic adenoma based on histopathology.[33]

Management of canalicular adenomas

Surgical excision, enucleation or limited extracapsular excisions have been used as treatment modalities in these tumors with success. Some surgeons have suggested that clinically benign neoplasms of the upper lip should be treated as mixed tumors and should be excised with a cuff of normal tissue surrounding the tumor.[33]

Ductal papilloma

Besides Warthin's tumor, benign papillary tumors of the salivary glands are rare. However there are three types with unique histopathologic features classified as sialadenoma papilleferum, inverted ductal papilloma and Intraductal papilloma.[34]

Sialadenoma papilleferum

This entity was first described by Abrams and Finck in 1969. It was termed sialadenoma papilleferum because of its histologic similarity to syringocystadenoma papilleferum of skin adnexal origin. According to cases registered in the AFIP registry, sialadenoma papilleferum constitutes only 0.1% of the epithelial salivary gland tumors.[34] However, Regezi et al have reported an incidence of 1.3%.[35]

Clinical features

The clinical presentation of this tumor is quite unique. Most of the salivary gland neoplasms present as a subsurface nodular swelling with smooth, intact mucosa or skin. However sialadenoma papilleferum presents as an exophytic, papillary surface lesion. It can be confused with squamous papilloma at presentation.

They mainly affect minor salivary glands of the oral or pharyngeal mucosa, most common site according to AFIP registry being posterior hard palate and soft palate. The junction of soft and hard palate is a common site with the tumor located on one side of the midline. The retromandibular trigone and buccal mucosa are less frequently involved where as gingiva, faucial pillars, upper lip and pharyngeal mucosa are rarely involved.

Size is usually subcentimetric. The tumor is asymptomatic and hence they are discovered mostly during routine oral examinations. Patients might feel these tumors as small growths on the mucosa with their tongues.

This tumor occurs at an average age of 56 years, cases being reported from 2 to 87 years. Male predilection is seen in the ratio of 1.5 to 1. However there is no racial predominance.

Gross pathology[34]

On gross examination the specimen reveals a round to oval, well circumscribed lesion of the surface mucosa. The lesion may be broad based or pedunculated. The surface of the tumor appears rough, pebbly, verrucous or papillary. It is often reddish. On cut section it gives a cauliflower appearance with circumscribed nodules of the tumor tissue extending below the level of the mucosa. Small cystic spaces might be seen on close visualization.

Histopathology[34]

On histological sections these tumors display both an exophytic and endophytic proliferation of the surface mucosa. The mucosal surface of the lesion is formed by many papillary projections of epithelial cells supported by cores of fibrovascular tissue which rise above the surface of the mucosa. The epithelial surface is covered by parakeratotic, acanthotic stratified squamous epithelium. At the junction of the normal mucosa the epithelium may have a pseudoepitheliomatous appearance with wide rounded rete ridges that push into the lamina propria. Normal mucosa may form a part of the stalk in cases of pedunculated tumors. It may form a lip or rolled border with more broad based tumors. The fibrovascular cores of papillary projections have a mild to intense, mixed inflammatory cell infiltrate of lymphocytes, plasma cells and neutrophils. Some exocytosis and intraepithelial microabscesses may be noted. Below the surface papillary projections the stratified squamous epithelium merges into ductal epithelium which lines branching, often tortuous duct like lumina that are contiguous with the interpapillary clefts of the surface stratified squamous epithelium. At the base of the lesion a proliferation of small ducts develops some of which may be cystically enlarged. There is no capsule around the proliferative ductal structures.

The ductal epithelium that lines the ducts, cysts and papillary folds usually comprises of double layer of cells. The luminal cells are composed of tall columnar cells and basilar cells are small cuboidal cells with a prominently eosinophilic cytoplasm. They resemble striated and interlobular excretory

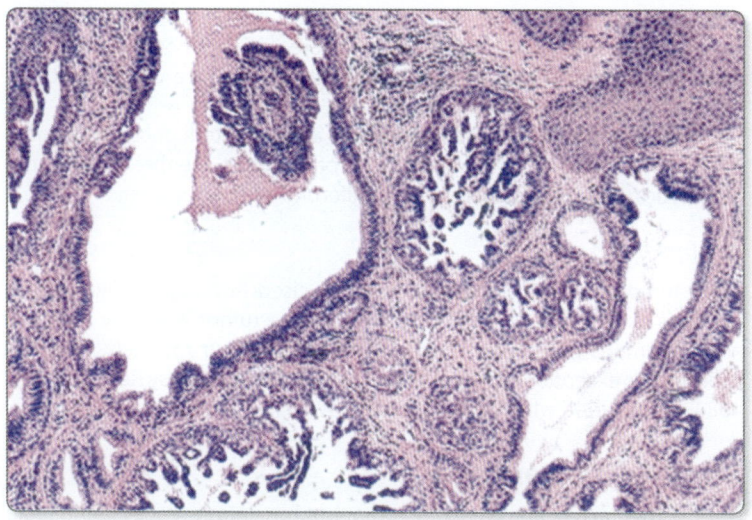

Figure 11.12 Photomicrograph of sialadenoma papilleferum (40X)
(*Source:* Ellis GL, Editor. Surgical pathology of the salivary glands)

duct cells. The cells of the glandular proliferations at the base of the tumor often have a deeply eosinophilic, oncocytic appearance. Scattered mucous cells may be seen which can be highlighted with mucicarine or periodic acid-schiff stain.

Differential diagnosis

Both the clinical and histopathologic features are similar to squamous papilloma. Clinically it may resemble a warty dyskeratoma or incipient verrucous carcinoma. However they can be ruled out on microscopic examination due to presence of ductal and glandular proliferations.

On histopathologic examination, due to the presence of mucous, squamous, ductal cells, and cystic structures along with absence of encapsulation it can be confused with mucoepidermoid carcinoma. However the gross appearance of exophytic and papillary growth in case of sialoadenoma papilleferum distinguishes it from mucoepidermoid carcinoma. The arrangement of the stratified squamous epithelium as caps on the papillary fronds of sialadenoma papilliferum is considerably different from the intermingling of epidermoid, mucous, and ductal cells that is seen in mucoepidermoid carcinoma.

In case there is marked pseudoepitheliomatous hyperplasia of the mucosal surface epithelium, it may be misdiagnosed as necrotizing sialometaplasia. However necrotizing sialometaplasia lacks the arborizing and papillary proliferation of ducts and the exophytic fronds covered by ductal and squamous epithelium, whereas sialadenoma papilliferum lacks the necrotizing lobules of salivary glands that are characteristic of necrotizing sialometaplasia.

Although the intraductal papilloma and inverted ductal papilloma share some features with sialadenoma papilliferum, neither exhibits the exophytic growth of sialadenoma papilliferum.

Treatment and prognosis

These tumors are typically small and easily excised. Although a salivary gland tumor is usually unsuspected clinically and the tumor is usually removed as a squamous papilloma, recurrence does not occur routinely. Thus the prognosis is exceptionally good. A palatal tumor reported by Rennie et al in 1984, has recurred which was treated by re-excision.[36]

Inverted ductal papilloma

Inverted ductal papilloma is a rare tumor but has unique readily identifiable histologic features. Inverted ductal papilloma was first described as an entity by White et al in 1982 when they reported four cases.[37]

Clinical features[34]

All reported cases have occurred in adults in the age range of 32 and 66 years. The mean age of occurrence is 50 years. There is no predilection for any particular sex. The sites usually involved are lower lip and buccal vestibular mucosa in descending order with occasional cases reported in upper lip, floor of mouth and soft palate.

It occurs as a firm, discrete nodule of 1–1.5 cm beneath the normal mucosa. In some cases a small surface pore may be contiguous with the tumor lumen. This tumor is asymptomatic.

Histopathology[34]

The tumor occurs within the terminal portion of a minor salivary gland excretory duct and therefore has some resemblance to sialadenoma papilliferum. However, the histopathologic features differ from those of sialadenoma papilliferum. The inverted ductal papilloma may produce bulging of the mucosal surface, but it does not extend above it like the papillary fronds of sialadenoma papilliferum.

Low magnification microscopic examination reveals a well-circumscribed tumor mass within the lamina propria that has an epidermoid appearance. Basaloid and squamoid cells are arranged in thick, bulbous proliferations that project in papillary configurations into a luminal cavity. They appear to fill the cavity and extend outwardly into the surrounding lamina propria. At the periphery, the tumor has a broad, well-demarcated, "pushing"

Surgical pathology of salivary gland neoplasms

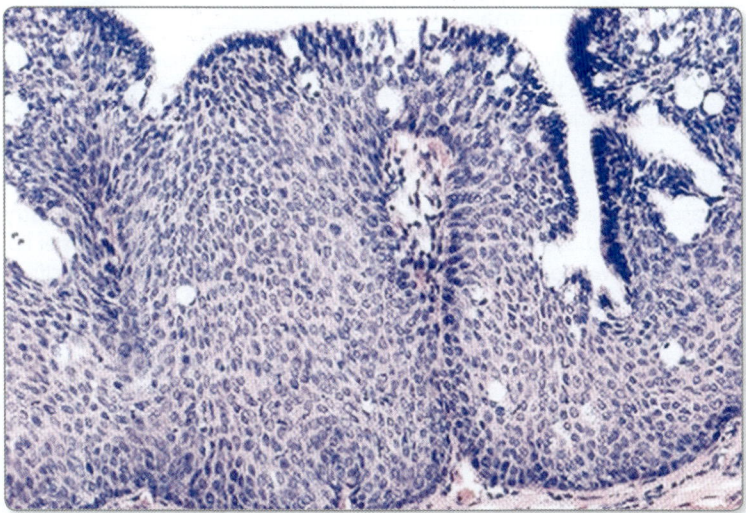

Figure 11.13 Photomicrograph of inverted ductal papilloma (40X) (*Source:* Ellis GL, Editor. Surgical pathology of the salivary glands)

interface with the connective tissue stroma of the lamina propria and the submucosa. There are no features of infiltration or invasion that might suggest malignancy. Because the tumor arises in the excretory duct, it is extra glandular, but if the excision is deep enough, there may be minor salivary gland lobules adjacent to or beneath the tumor.

The lumen of the tumor is often narrow and branching as a result of the proliferation of tumor cells in broad papillae into the lumen. In some tumors, the lumen communicates by a constricted opening with the exterior of the mucosal surface. The stratified squamous epithelium of the mucosal epithelium forms a lip at this opening and is contiguous with the tumor epithelium.

High-magnification microscopy reveals several cell types within this neoplastic proliferation. The bulk of the tumor is composed of basaloid or immature epidermoid cells. The luminal surface of the papillary proliferation is often covered by columnar or cuboidal, ductlike cells that have eosinophilic cytoplasm. Interspersed among these ductal cells may be mucous cells that stain positively with periodic acid-Schiff and mucicarmine stains. Within the tumor epithelium, small microcysts that contain a mucinous material usually are evident.

Treatment and prognosis

It is treated by simple surgical excision as it is not known to recur.

Intraductal papilloma

Reports of this salivary gland tumor are rare in English scientific literature not only because this tumor is uncommon but also because the definition of this tumor varies considerably in literature.

Clinical features[34]

24 cases of intraductal papilloma are registered in the salivary gland registry of the AFIP. Of these 24 tumors, 10 occurred in the lips; four in the upper lip, five in the lower lip, and one in the upper or lower lip that is not specified. Other sites of occurrence, in descending order of frequency, were the palate, the buccal mucosa, the parotid gland duct, and the submandibular gland duct. If found in the minor salivary glands, these tumors present as asymptomatic, submucosal swellings that vary in size from less than 1 to 1.5 cm. The ages of patients range from 29 to 77 years, with a mean age of 54 years. Men and women are equally affected.

Gross pathology[34]

Sections of the gross specimen show a well circumscribed cyst with a lumen that is partially or completely filled with friable tissue that extends from the wall of the cyst.

Histopathology[34]

The papilloma appears to arise in the duct system more distant from the mucosal surface than from where the inverted ductal papilloma arises. The proliferating epithelium is characteristic of the ductal epithelium in this location. The cyst wall is lined by a single or double layer of cuboidal and columnar cells. Extending into the cyst lumen is several to numerous papillary fronds that have thin fibrovascular cores. In cross-sections, the papillary fronds may have a complex branching structure that creates an appearance of islands of tumor that are floating in the cyst lumen. The papillary projections are covered by the same cuboidal and columnar ductal epithelium. Mucous cells may be interspersed among the ductal cells, or as in the tumor described by Kerpel and coworkers, they may predominate.[38] There is no proliferation of epithelium into or beyond the cyst wall. Within the connective tissue of the cyst wall, minimal to moderate inflammatory cell infiltrates may be present.

Treatment and prognosis

Excision is curative, and these tumors are not known to recur. In case the tumors are small, all types of papillomas of the minor salivary glands, including intraductal, inverted, and sialadenoma papilliferum, can be excised in the dental office or the clinic under local anesthesia.[34]

Malignant tumors of salivary glands

Malignant tumors comprise only 3 percent of all head and neck tumors and demonstrate an unpredictable clinical course marked by frequent locoregional failure and distant metastasis, often occurring years after diagnosis.[39]

Mucoepidermoid carcinoma

Mucoepidermoid carcinoma is the most common malignant salivary gland neoplasm. Only the benign pleomorphic adenoma has a higher incidence rate than mucoepidermoid carcinoma. It is the second most common malignancy (after ACC) of the sub-mandibular and minor salivary glands. Mucoepidermoid carcinoma constitutes approximately 5–12% of salivary gland tumors[40] and 35% of salivary gland malignancy. 80% to 90% of mucoepidermoid carcinomas occur in the parotid gland. As its name implies, mucoepidermoid carcinoma includes two major elements; viz: mucin-producing cells and epithelial cells of the epidermoid variety. These two different cells may originate from an intermediate cell, which is also present in mucoepidermoid carcinoma. This dual cell type forms the basis of classifying this tumor into a three-tiered histologic grading system: Grade I (low grade) are well differentiated, grade II (intermediate grade) are moderately differentiated, and grade III (high grade) are poorly differentiated tumors.

The term 'mucoepidermoid tumor' was first used by Stewart, Foote and Becker in 1945.[41] However, in 1939, De and Tribedi had already mentioned regarding this tumor as a mixed epidermoid and mucous secreting carcinoma of the parotid gland.

Clinical features

Mucoepidermoid carcinoma is the most common malignant salivary gland neoplasm. Spiro et al have reported 15.7 percent of all benign and malignant salivary gland tumors and 34 percent of the malignant salivary gland tumors to be mucoepidermoid carcinomas.[41] Eveson and Cawson have reported that only 2.1 percent of salivary gland tumors in their study were mucoepidermoid carcinomas, and Thackray and Lucas have reported only a slightly higher figure. Hence there could be a difference in the relative frequency of this neoplasm among American, English, and possibly other Western European populations and thus may reflect a true geographic variation.[41]

Mucoepidermoid carcinomas show a relatively uniform age distribution between, the second and eighth decades of life. Occurrence in the first decade is extremely rare, but there is a rapid rise in incidence in the second decade. Mucoepidermoid carcinoma is the most common malignant salivary gland tumor in patients under 20 years of age.[42] The mean age of males and females for all cases is nearly identical. Some variation in the mean age of males and females dependent on the anatomic location is evident.[41]

Overall, females are affected slightly more often than males. The gender difference is most pronounced for patients with lesions of the tongue and retromolar areas; females make up over 80 and 76 percent of these patients, respectively.[41]

Incidence of mucoepidermoid carcinoma in the minor glands is 2-3 times higher than major salivary glands.[41,45] However according to AFIP registry, 54 percent of all mucoepidermoid carcinomas occur in the major salivary glands, and most of the remaining 46 percent arise from the intraoral minor salivary glands. Nearly 47 percent of all cases occurred in the parotid glands according to AFIP registry.[41] According to few studies as many as two-thirds of all mucoepidermoid carcinomas occur in the parotid gland.[43]

The hard and soft palates account for nearly 18 percent of all mucoepidermoid carcinomas, and these tumors account for 44 percent of all malignant salivary gland tumors that involve these sites. The cheek, the lips, the floor of the mouth, and the retromolar region together constitute nearly another 18 percent of all cases. The lower lip is involved about three times more often than the upper lip although the lower lip is much less commonly affected than the upper lip by salivary gland tumors of other types.[41,44] The exact site of most of the tumors of the tongue occurred at the base, the most common area for malignant salivary gland tumors of the tongue regardless of histologic type.[45]

It occurs as a painless solitary enlargement of the body or tail of the parotid or the submandibular region. Its duration usually averages less than 1 year. However they could be of a longer duration too. Tumors of 20 years and 40 years duration have also been reported in literature.[43] Growth of the tumor sometimes extends over a period of months or years, simulating the appearance of a mucocele (Gorlin, 1985), retention cyst or fibroma, especially in the region of minor salivary glands.[40] Cases with accelerated growth after a period of quiescence have been reported, thus suggestive that the biologic nature of the tumor may change with time.

The tumor clinically is well circumscribed and movable, and may mimic a mixed tumor **(Figure 11.14)**. Pain, facial paralysis, and fixation to the overlying skin are not common but when present are usually suggestive of high-grade lesions. Facial nerve palsy occurs most often with high-grade mucoepidermoid carcinomas.[41]

Multinodularity is rarely noted in the tumor. The size of most parotid tumors is between 1 and 4 cm in diameter, but patients may present with much larger tumors if they delay seeking medical advice. Many minor salivary

Surgical pathology of salivary gland neoplasms   133

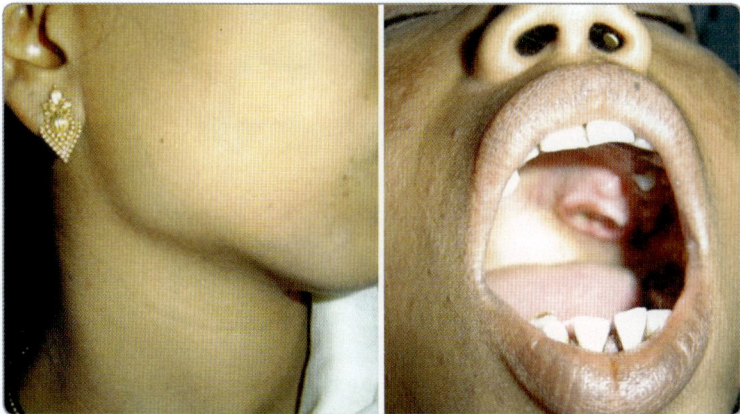

Figure 11.14 Mucoepidermoid carcinoma of submandibular gland and minor gland of palate

gland mucoepidermoid carcinomas are discovered incidentally during a routine dental examination. The clinical presentation of mucoepidermoid carcinomas of the minor salivary glands is protean and defies concise description. Many lesions present as a bluish or red-purple, fluctuant, smoothsurfaced mass that is often clinically mistaken for a mucocele. Clinical diagnosis of hemangioma or nevus may be made due to magenta color of several tumors. Mucus may be discharged through a small opening on the mucosal surface leading to misinterpretation as a draining dental abscess by the examining doctor. Focal erythema or even ecchymosis may be seen. Some mucoepidermoid carcinomas have a granular or papillary surface and are thought to be papillomas or verrucous carcinomas. Few occur as hard masses that may be clinically interpreted as osteomas or tori. Large lesions at the base of the tongue or in the oropharynx may cause dysphagia.

Ulceration is associated with lesions which, in most cases, have an aggressive clinical course. Numbness of teeth may occur when bone is involved. Cupping of bone, most often of the hard palate, is seen often enough. Hence thorough radiographic evaluation of any mucoepidermoid carcinoma that involves mucosa overlying bone should be performed.

Gross pathology[41]

On macroscopic examination, most mucoepidermoid carcinomas are relatively well circumscribed. They may appear at least partially encapsulated and, rarely, complete encapsulation is noted. Accurate delimitation of the borders may be difficult or impossible to determine by gross inspection. The cut surface is usually firm and pinkish or yellowish tan.

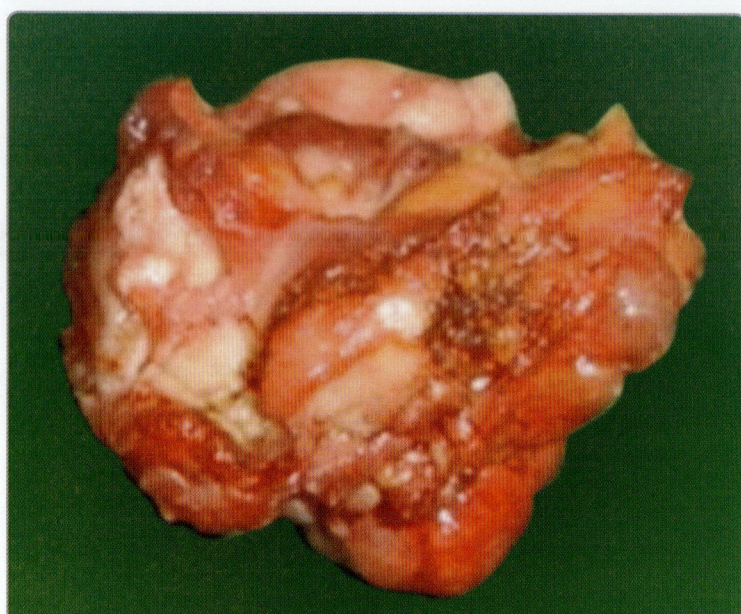

Figure 11.15 Cut section of mucoepidermoid carcinoma

Extreme induration is occasionally present. Cyst formation may be readily evident, but the prominence of this element varies. The majority of the cut surface may be cystic or, there may be such haphazard distribution of the cysts that only a fraction of the entire surface is cystic. The cystic spaces contain viscid, translucent mucoid material that may be blood tinged. Focal hemorrhage is sometimes present and may be striking, particularly if a previous invasive procedure, such as an incisional biopsy or fine-needle aspiration, has been performed.

Histopathology[41]

Mucoepidermoid carcinomas are characterized histologically by the presence of a variety of cell types and growth patterns, both of which form the basis for recognition and grading. Grading is based on the presence or absence of particular cell types or growth patterns in addition to the proportion of each element relative to the other. The recognition of this tumor involves identification of mucous, epidermoid, intermediate, columnar, or clear cells, each proliferating alone or in many different combinations, in a cystic or solid pattern. Mucous cells are those cells that contain epithelial mucin.

Surgical pathology of salivary gland neoplasms

Special stains are required to verify identification of mucous cells in some mucoepidermoid carcinomas. Neoplastic mucous cells have abundant, pale, foamy cytoplasm, and are usually relatively large, and may assume round, cuboidal, ovoid, columnar, or goblet appearance. These foamy mucous cells often occur in small clusters or line a cystic space into which mucin is deposited. In many instances, mucous cells are scattered singly, vastly outnumbered by other cell types or, in high-grade lesions, they may be extremely rare. Large edematous squamoid cells may be present that have pale, eosinophilic, granular cytoplasm. They may be misinterpreted as mucous cells. Histochemical verification of the epithelial mucin which stains positively for mucicarmine and periodic acid-Schiff and is resistant to diastase digestion is useful. Tumors with predominant mucous cells are found more commonly in the minor salivary glands. Tumor cells that are often more important than mucous cells for the recognition of mucoepidermoid carcinomas are a group of highly prolific, basaloid cells, referred to as intermediate cells. Intermediate cells demonstrate gradual transitions in sizes from small basal cells, which are slightly larger than lymphocytes and have little to no discernible cytoplasm; to cells having a wide rim of cytoplasm sometimes more pronounced toward one end of the cell; and finally, to cells with ample, evenly distributed cytoplasm. When enlargement of intermediate cells occurs to a size more than two to three times the size of basaloid cells, they are referred to as epidermoid cells. There is no clear distinction between the large intermediate cells and the epidermoid cells. The two cell types are often amalgamated into solid tumor islands, and they become very difficult to distinguish from one another. The cytoplasmic borders of intermediate cells are sometimes sharply demarcated, notably so in areas where cells are less cohesive; however, often the cells have a more syncytial arrangement in which individual borders can be appreciated only with difficulty. As basaloid cells mature, their nuclei enlarge, although this enlargement is proportionately smaller than their cytoplasmic increase, and the original condensed nuclear chromatin becomes more vesicular.

Epidermoid cells, together with intermediate and mucous cells, line cystic spaces or form solid masses. The epidermoid or squamous cell zones may be sharply demarcated from the intermediate cells, or they may blend imperceptibly with other cells from which they have apparently originated. Squamous cells only occasionally form keratin pearls or become individually keratinized, but some degree of stratification is normally evident. Clear cells are large and polygonal and have sharply defined cytoplasmic borders. They morphologically resemble squamous cells, and transition from one of these cell types to the other is sometimes obvious. Clear cells may dominate large areas of the tumor, which complicates interpretation. Infrequently these cells contain abundant, demonstrable mucin, but in most clear cells, only traces are seen focally. Examination of multiple sections of predominantly clear cell tumors often discloses the more characteristic blend of mucous, intermediate, and epidermoid cells and reveals the true nature of the tumor.

Grading of mucoepidermoid carcinoma

It has been stated that features such as clinical staging and histological grading correlate with the clinical behavior of mucoepidermoid carcinoma in spite of using various criteria for grading of the tumors such as invasion of adjacent structures, cystic or solid growth pattern, types of cellularity participating in the neoplastic process and pleomorphism, immunohistochemical demonstration of proteins both in neoplastic and non-neoplastic cells of affected glands and mitotic activity.[40]

Grading mucoepidermoid carcinomas is subjective. Mucoepidermoid carcinomas have been classified in to three grades based on their histopathological findings. Grade I tumors show a predominance of mucus-secreting cells and well-differentiated epidermoid cells. Grade III tumors show few or no mucus-producing cells and poorly differentiated epidermoid cells. This variety can sometimes be mistaken for poorly differentiated squamous cell carcinoma. In such cases, meticulous search for any mucus-producing cells by a thorough microscopic examination, and in some cases, with the use of special stains for mucin, will usually provide the diagnosis of mucoepidermoid carcinomas.

The grading criteria originally conceived by Foote and Frazel which was considered as most useful most often included the following:
1. The degree of cyst formation as opposed to solid growth.
2. The proportion of cell types.
3. The presence or absence of cytomorphologic atypia.

In 1968, Jakobsson and colleagues disregarded the original criteria and used the presence of invasion as the only criterion for determining low and high grades; however, their meaning of "invasion" was not defined. Later, Healey and coworkers considered the "extent" of invasiveness in addition to the simultaneous evaluation of cyst formation, cellular anaplasia, and mitotic activity. In 1984, Acetta and coworkers used the original criteria in conjunction with one of three defined patterns of invasion: (1) borders with partial encapsulation or good circumscription, (2) broad pushing borders with limited invasion, and (3) infiltrative growth with permeation into surrounding tissue. These authors concluded that the only finding common to all tumors that metastasized was an infiltrating border. Most investigators have considered the degree of cellular maturation, cellularity, and mitotic figures important to grading.

The term "invasion" in context to grading of mucoepidermoid carcinomas refers to the permeation of connective tissue by small cords and islands of tumor and individual tumor cells. Nearly all mucoepidermoid carcinomas are poorly circumscribed and infiltrative. However some high-grade tumors demonstrate broad, pushing borders that are more typical of low-grade tumors. Since minor salivary glands are normally located within fibrous connective tissue or skeletal muscle, tumors that originate from these glands often falsely appear extensively infiltrative.

Low grade mucoepidermoid carcinoma

The hallmark of low-grade lesions is prominent cystic structure and this feature is accompanied by the presence of numerous, mature cellular elements, including mucous cells and often abundant extra cellular mucin. The cysts may infiltrate adjacent salivary gland parenchyma and connective tissue. However, neural invasion is not normally seen in low-grade tumors. In case it is present, it is a cause of concern and additional sections should be reviewed. The linings of the cysts vary in thickness and in cellular composition, but typically, a mixture of cell types, one to three cells thick, is evident. Uniformly thin layer of cuboidal cells may line large cystic spaces, but their continuity is interrupted focally by solid proliferations of other cell types. A mixture of mucous, intermediate, and epidermoid cells is seen routinely. Mucous cells are more prevalent in low-grade than in high-grade tumors. Small gland like formations may have a central lumen that is filled with mucus, and mucus also fills many of the large, cystic spaces. These often rupture, spill their contents into adjacent tissues and frequently incite an inflammatory reaction. This increases the possibility

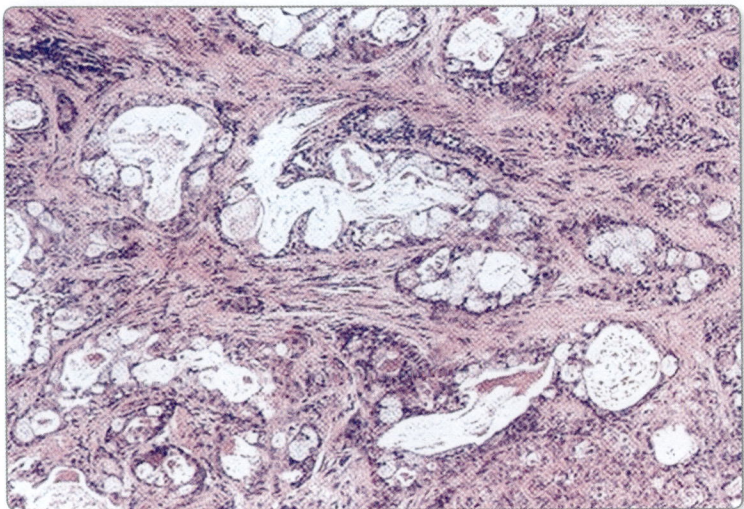

Figure 11.16 Photomicrograph of low-grade mucoepidermoid carcinoma (40X)
(*Source:* Ellis GL, Editor. Surgical pathology of the salivary glands)

for tumor cells to spread more easily and may also complicate complete surgical excision. Luminal outgrowths of cyst lining epithelium vary from focal excrescences to well-formed papillary projections. Squamous cells lining cystic spaces may be evident, and close examination may reveal intercellular bridges. Solid islands or cords of cells are often present, but large sheet like proliferations are not seen in low-grade tumors. The size, shape, and staining characteristics of all cell types are uniform; mitoses are extremely rare or absent.

Intermediate grade mucoepidermoid carcinoma

Intermediate-grade tumors show quantitative and qualitative differences of the cystic elements. The cysts constitute a much smaller proportion of the entire tumor mass because they are fewer in number and are smaller than those seen in low-grade lesions. The cellular composition typically shows a predominance of intermediate cells, often with scattered mucous cells and zones of epidermoid cells, forming large, solid islands of tumor. Squamous cells may rarely demonstrate keratin pearl formation. Mucous cells are usually readily evident, and mucin stains reveal numerous additional cells that stain positively for mucin. Nuclear atypia is not a necessary feature, but it may be focally evident. Mitotic figures are quite rare, but nucleoli are noted more often in intermediate-grade lesions than in low-grade lesions. The distinction between the low and the intermediate grades is primarily

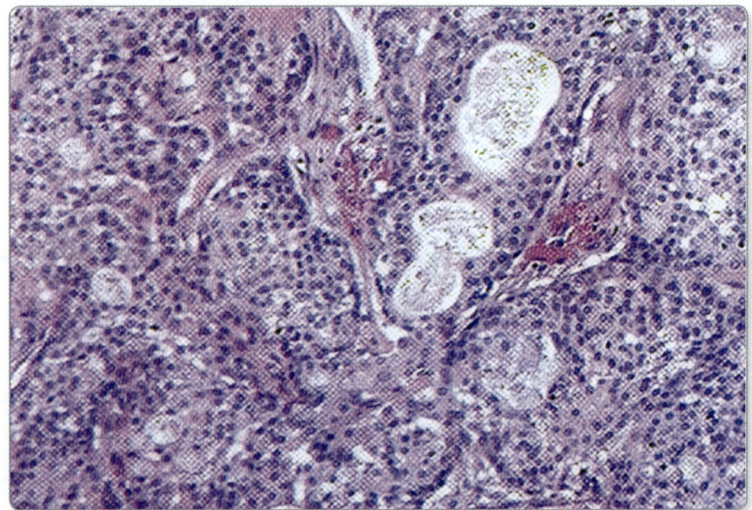

Figure 11.17 Photomicrograph of intermediate-grade mucoepidermoid carcinoma (40X)
(*Source:* Ellis GL, Editor. Surgical pathology of the salivary glands)

based on the relative proportion of the cystic and solid cellular areas and the predominance of intermediate and epidermoid cells.

High grade mucoepidermoid carcinoma

They are characterized by nearly solid cellular proliferations of epidermoid and intermediate cells, which display a noticeable degree of cytologic atypia. The nuclear-cytoplasmic ratio of many cells is altered. Also, nucleoli are prominent, and mitoses may be numerous. High-grade mucoepidermoid carcinomas may show at least two different patterns. The first resembles a moderately differentiated squamous cell carcinoma because of a diffuse proliferation of epidermoid cells which have a moderate degree of cellular pleomorphism. The presence of glandular or small cystic structures can help separate high-grade mucoepidermoid carcinoma from squamous cell carcinoma but, when absent, histochemical demonstration of cells that test positive for mucin can also be diagnostic. The second pattern is characterized by a variety of cell types that are most often dominated by intermediate cells, but mucous, epidermoid, and squamous cells are often seen. Many cells demonstrate a moderate degree of anaplasia. The solid, hypercellular proliferation of morphologically abnormal cells, form a hallmark of the high-grade tumors. Sufficient cellular pleomorphism is present to allow distinction from low and intermediate-grade tumors, and with either pattern, mitotic activity is usually prominent.

Management of mucoepidermoid carcinoma

Complete surgical excision is the treatment of choice for mucoepidermoid carcinomas. Adequate excision is important in all grades of tumors. Prognosis of mucoepidermoid carcinomas is a function of the histological grade, adequacy of excision and clinical staging. The immunohistochemical study of Ki-67 expression may provide additional prognostic information for this tumor.[46]

Irrespective of morphological sub-typing, radical resection of the primary tumor has to be attempted in all patients.[40] In case of stage I and stage II mucoepidermoid carcinomas of the parotid gland conservative excision with preservation of the facial nerve, if possible, is recommended. The affected submandibular gland should be removed entirely. Radical neck dissection is performed in patients with clinical evidence of cervical node metastasis and is considered in any patient with a T3 lesion. Elective lymphadenectomy in patients with high grade lesions but no apparent nodal involvement is not routinely practiced. In the past, patients with facial nerve paralysis were considered incurable, but recent studies have shown that this presentation does not necessarily signify incurable disease. Patients were treated by reducing the nerve back to the histologically tumor-negative nerve trunk, and in some cases, this was followed by postoperative radiation. The 5-year disease-free rate in patients receiving this aggressive treatment was about 60 percent.[41]

Treatment of minor salivary gland mucoepidermoid carcinomas is also primarily surgical. Wide surgical excision is recommended, with the goal of ensuring tumor, free margins.[47] The wound is often left open to heal secondarily. If the tumor erodes or invades underlying bone, a portion of the mandible or maxilla should be excised to obtain a margin free of tumor. Mucoepidermoid carcinoma of the retromolar mucosa often involves bone; therefore, this site, in particular, should be evaluated radiographically prior to surgery.

Optimal treatment of lesions of the hard palate remains controversial. Olsen and coworkers state that regardless of tumor grade or size, partial maxillectomy should be accomplished.[47] Tran and colleagues advocate radical palatectomy and postoperative radiation therapy for high-grade tumors or if margins are questionable.[48] Melrose and co-investigators believe that treatment involving local excision with a modest margin of clinically normal tissue or, if there is evidence of bone destruction, block removal of underlying bone is adequate for well-differentiated tumors.[41] For small low grade tumors in the absence of bone involvement, wide excision down to periosteum with 1- or 2-cm tumor-free lateral margins is adequate therapy.[41] High-grade and advanced stage tumors must be treated aggressively at any site. Enucleation of these high-grade lesions is to be avoided to gain a more favorable outcome and reduce recurrences. Indications for neck dissection are similar to those for the major salivary glands, but primary tumors of the tongue are of particular concern, especially lesions larger than 2 cm. In these cases, neck dissection, followed by resection of the primary tumor through the mandible, should be performed.[47] Lymph node dissection may also be indicated if lymphadenopathy is present in cases of high-grade tumors from any site and in cases with lesions larger than 4 cm.

Mucoepidermoid carcinoma is very rare in the pediatric age group. Treatment involves surgical removal of the tumor plus radiotherapy, according to histologic staging. Mucoepidermoid carcinoma has a good prognosis in young patients. The survival rate does not differ in the subgroup of patients with mucoepidermoid carcinoma as a secondary tumor.[49]

Radiotherapy

In 1970, Jakobsson and Eneroth considered mucoepidermoid carcinoma as one of the types of salivary gland cancer that was not radiosensitive, but the radiation doses delivered at that time are low if compared to those used today.[41] Recently higher dose therapeutic radiation has been shown to be beneficial for high-grade and advanced stage tumors and for those tumors that involve the facial nerve.[50]

Surgical pathology of salivary gland neoplasms   141

There has been a divided opinion regarding postoperative radiotherapy for malignant tumors affecting the parotid gland. Tran and colleagues concluded that adjuvant radiation therapy offered no increase in local control or survival among patients who had surgical excision with margins free of tumor. They noted that radiation may improve local control and survival if residual disease is found at the surgical margins in a patient no longer amenable to surgery, but that radiation therapy was not an adequate substitute for leaving clear surgical margins.[51] The data from studies by Fu and colleagues, King and Fletcher, Chung and coworkers, and Mc-Naney and coinvestigators indicated that 5,000 to 7,000 rad (50 to 70 Gy) of postoperative irradiation given over 5 to 6 weeks may improve the local control rate for cases with gross or microscopic disease at the margins of resection.[41] There is some evidence that fast neutron radiotherapy may have more success than conventional photon therapy, especially for tumors in advanced stages. Catterall M, Errington RD in 1987 have reported a 74 percent local control rate for patients with unresectable tumors with facial nerve involvement, and some patients maintained function of the facial nerve.[41]

Recurrence, metastasis and prognosis

The overall recurrence rate of mucoepidermoid carcinomas is approximately 25%. However there is a gross variance in individual recurrence rates of different grades of mucoepidermoid tumors.[41]

In a study by Thorvaldsson and colleagues, they have reported a recurrence rate of 10% for low-grade lesions and 74% recurrence for high-grade lesions. Patients are more likely to have recurrence if the margins of resection are positive, regardless of grade.[52] Although most tumors that recur do so within one year of therapy, several cases of low- and intermediate–grade tumors recorded in AFIP registry have recurred or were reactivated after longer intervals. Similar delayed recurrences have also been noted by Spiro and Healey in their respective studies.[41]

The rates of both regional and distant metastases are influenced by the histologic grade, the clinical stage, and the specific site of origin. In a study by Spiro et al, metastases to regional lymph nodes appeared to be more frequent from submandibular tumors than from other major or minor gland sites. Although cervical metastases from the minor glands were usually not appreciated at the time of diagnosis, they also noted that over the course of the disease the parotid and minor glands had similar incidences of metastases. Distant metastases, however, occur less often with lesions of minor glands than with those of the parotid or submandibular glands. The distant sites most often involved are the lung, the skeleton, and the brain. No site is spared, however, and we have seen many high-grade tumors that disseminated widely throughout the body. Involvement of the intra parotid lymph nodes is much less significant than regional or distant metastasis.[53]

Survival is closely related to the clinical stage and the histologic grade. Although staging and grading are inter-related, they appear to work independently of each other. Grade I lesions behave less aggressively than grade III lesions, regardless of stage, and conversely, a lower stage lesion has a better prognosis than stage III or IV lesions, regardless of grade. Hence the pathologist and the surgeon together must consider both the grade and the stage when determining treatment and prognosis.

Other factors reported to influence prognosis are the age and the sex of the patient and the site of involvement. Better survival is seen among younger patients and among females. Conley and Tinsley in 1985 have concluded that the probability of death for children with this tumor is essentially zero. However other investigators have reported aggressive or fatal cases in young patients. Hence the need for thorough tumor removal, even in the younger population, need not be overemphasized. In a study by O'Brien et al, they have concluded that the prognosis for patients over the age of 60 years, regardless of other factors, is significantly worse than that for younger patients.[54] Tumors in the submandibular gland and in the base of the tongue generally have a poorer outlook than those at other major and minor salivary gland sites. Also invasion into bone signifies a poorer prognosis. Death from low-grade tumors is extremely rare, and in case of intermediate-grade and high-grade tumors it has been shown that most deaths occur before 10th year after initial diagnosis. There is a decrease in the death rate between eight and tenth year.[41]

Adenoid cystic carcinoma

Adenoid cystic carcinoma is an aggressive tumor of the head and neck region which occurs primarily in the major salivary glands and relatively frequently in the oral accessory salivary glands, particularly the palate. Since 1856, since it was first defined, it was falsely considered to be a benign tumor. Today it is recognized as a highly aggressive, destructive and clinically unpredictable tumor of the head and neck region.[55]

Theodor Billroth initially described this tumor and suggested that it be called cylindroma in 1856.[56] In 1945, Bauer and Fox suggested use of the term adenomyoepithelioma because the lesion was histogenetically derived from intercalated duct and myoepithelial cells. Dockerty and Mayo used the designation adenocarcinoma, cylindroma type. Foote and Frazell proposed the currently accepted term adenoid cystic carcinoma in their classic paper in 1953 and in their fascicle on major salivary gland tumors in 1954.

Clinical features[56]

Adenoid cystic carcinoma occurs most often in adults in the fifth, sixth, and seventh decades of life. Although the tumor is uncommon in young persons, occasional cases are encountered in the first 2 decades of life. Most series show an equal distribution of cases between both the sexes.

The most frequent locations of the tumor are the parotid, submandibular and palatal salivary glands.[57] They are only rarely observed in the sublingual gland.[56] However, Spiro and colleagues have reported that, only 1.6. percent of all parotid tumors are adenoid cystic carcinomas.[58] Eneroth reported a comparable rate of occurrence of 2.2 percent.[59] Eneroth and Hjertman found that 12 percent of all submandibular salivary glands to be ACC.[56] Relative to the sublingual glands, adenoid cystic carcinomas account for 40 percent of the tumors in this particular gland.[60] All reported series reflect the relatively frequent occurrence of adenoid cystic carcinoma in the minor salivary glands, particularly the palate. Although 42.5 percent of adenoid cystic carcinomas occurred in the minor glands, 20.5 percent were in the palate. In addition it is also found in other intraoral sites, viz tongue. Adenoid cystic carcinoma appears to be the third most common malignancy of the tongue; it is exceeded in frequency of occurrence only by epidermoid and mucoepidermoid carcinomas. Adenoid cystic carcinoma of the salivary glands of the buccal mucosa is also encountered frequently.[56]

Typically, adenoid cystic carcinoma is apparent in the major salivary glands as a swelling or as a mass. The tumor grows slowly; patients may be aware of the lesion for months and even years in some instances. Pain and tenderness generally occur during the course of tumor growth. Fixation to skin and to surrounding deeper structures develops in the later stages of tumor growth. An ominous feature of adenoid cystic carcinoma of the parotid gland as well as of other malignant salivary gland[61] neoplasms in this location is paralysis of the facial nerve. Adenoid cystic carcinoma of the intraoral accessory salivary glands presents typically as a swelling or mass. Pain is a variable finding, particularly in the early stages of development. As tumor growth progresses, pain and ulceration develop. Symptoms of facial pain and swelling characterize adenoid cystic carcinoma of the maxillary antrum, but these symptoms are not specific for this particular tumor. Radiographic examination is valuable in assessing the extent of osseous destruc-tion. Symptoms may have been present for months or years and are generally of longer duration than those associated with squamous carcinoma, which is the most frequent malignancy of this location. Adenoid cystic carcinomas of the nasal cavity and ear canal produce symptoms of obstruction and deafness, respectively.

Gross pathology[56]

Adenoid cystic carcinoma usually presents as a fairly well-defined mass within the, substance of the involved gland. On cut section, the tumor lacks encapsulation, although it may appear to be demarcated from the surrounding salivary gland tissue. Close inspection typically shows infiltration into the surrounding parenchymal tissue. The tumor is firm, white, or grayish-white and is not usually "cystic." Grossly observable "cystic" zones are uncommon, as are areas of hemorrhage.

Histopathology[56]

Adenoid cystic carcinoma has varied microscopic patterns. The actual cells that form these "patterns" are remarkably uniform in size, shape, and staining qualities. Thus, the tumor is composed of isomorphic cells that are arranged in various morphologic patterns. Depending on the relative prominence of these morphologic patterns, adenoid cystic carcinoma is seen to exist in: (1) The cribriform pattern, (2) The tubular pattern, and (3) The solid pattern.

Cribriform type

The cribriform pattern is the most important and most recognized microscopic type. The tumor cells are arranged in the so-called "Swiss cheese" configuration. The tumor cells are characterized by dark, deeply basophilic nuclei and scanty cytoplasm.

Nucleoli are seldom observed, and division figures are rarely encountered. The cells are arranged in nests of variable size and shape that contain many circular or ovoid spaces; these spaces impart the Swiss cheese pattern. The spaces may contain either a faintly basophilic mucinous substance or hyalinized eosinophilic zones. Other microscopic fields may show cords of the same isomorphic tumor cells within the hyalinized material. Both such fields may occur concomitantly in the same tumor field. The stroma of the tumor is typically fibrous; however, at times, it may be somewhat hyalinized.

Tubular type

The second major microscopic pattern of adenoid cystic carcinoma is the tubular type. The tumor cells are identical to those observed in the cribriform pattern; however, the arrangement of these cells is different. Single ductal structures are formed by layers of the isomorphic cells. In longitudinal section these ductal structures are viewed as ducts or tubules, a feature that is responsible for the designation of this histologic pattern. It is obvious that the ducts or tubules in cross-section and in longitudinal section may be viewed in the same tumor. The lumina may contain a mucinous substance that is faintly eosinophilic. This material typically stains positively

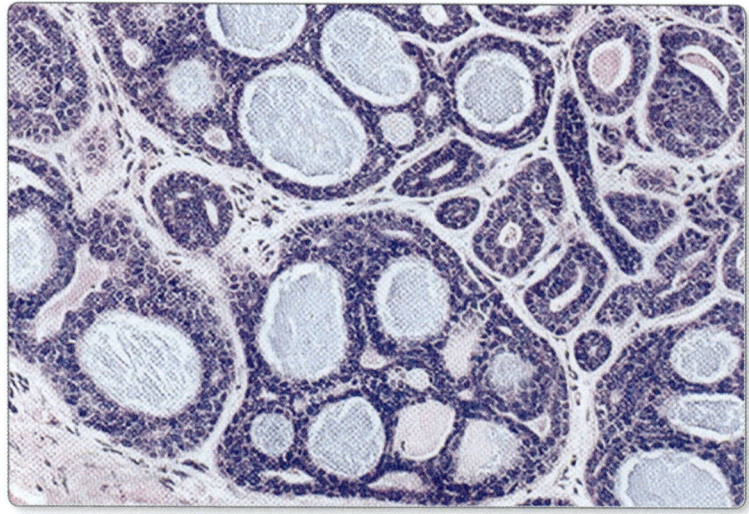

Figure 11.18 Photomicrograph of cribriform type adenoid cystic carcinoma (40X)
(*Source:* Ellis GL, Editor. Surgical pathology of the salivary glands)

with periodic acid-Schiff (PAS) stain before and after diastase digestion. Cribriform areas may coexist with the tubular pattern, and transitions may be observed.

Solid type

The third major microscopic pattern of adenoid cystic carcinoma is the solid type. The isomorphic tumor cells characteristic of the cribriform and tubular types are arranged in nests or sheets of varying size and shape. There is no, or only a minimal, tendency to form the circular or ovoid spaces that characterize the cribriform type, and no ducts or tubular structures like those observed in the tubular type are formed. Occasionally, areas of necrosis may be found centrally within some of the solid nests. In addition to foci of necrosis, cellular pleomorphism and mitoses may be observed in this pattern, which are features that are not usually found in the other patterns of adenoid cystic carcinoma.

However, most adenoid cystic carcinomas do not occur in "pure" cribriform, tubular, or solid types but all three patterns can be observed in the majority of tumors. Generally, tumors are classified according to the histologic pattern that predominates. A major microscopic feature in most adenoid cystic carcinomas is the propensity for the tumor to involve peripheral nerves. This neurotropic tendency has been reported to occur in 20 to 80% of the patients.[7] The tumor not only invests the perineural space

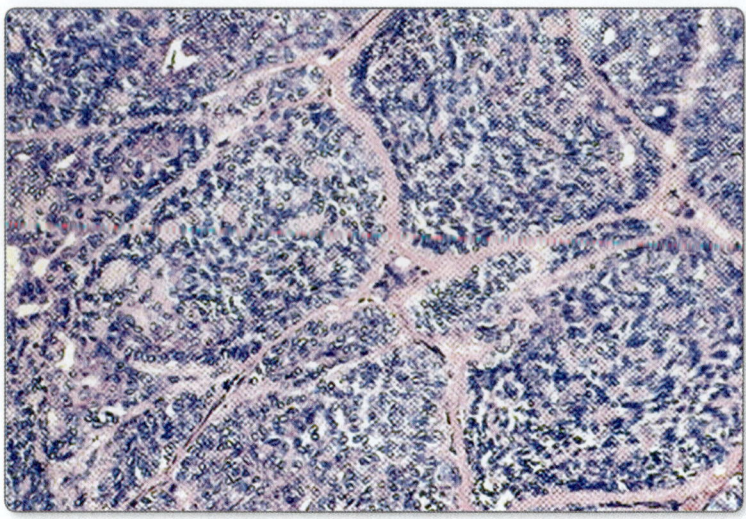

Figure 11.19 Photomicrograph of cribriform type adenoid cystic carcinoma (40X) (*Source:* Ellis GL, Editor. Surgical pathology of the salivary glands)

but also actual neural invasion can be observed. Neurovascular structures are involved less commonly. The older concept of perineural lymphatics is considered obsolete today. Instead it is considered to be a potential anatomic space composed of the loosely arranged perineural tissues. Although perineural invasion is characteristic of adenoid cystic carcinoma, it is not unique to the tumor. Polymorphous low-grade adenocarcinoma and salivary duct carcinoma, in particular, have shown a propensity for perineural involvement.[56,62]

Management of adenoid cystic carcinoma

It is known that local control and distant hematogenous metastasis are major problems in the management of adenoid cystic carcinoma. It has high likelihood of metastasis to the regional lymph nodes. They have a high propensity for perineural spread and hence they should also be managed along the path of cranial nerve at risk for involvement.[62] The slow biologic growth of adenoid cystic carcinoma coupled with metastasis late in the course of the disease results in relatively favorable 5-year survival rates. However, the long-term outlook for survival and cure is far less favorable.

Salivary gland adenoid cystic carcinoma has a dismal ultimate prognosis for cure, although long-term survivors, even with persistent disease, are not uncommon. Factors that indicate a poor prognosis include failure of local disease control at the initial surgical procedure, a solid pattern histologically, recurrent disease and distant metastasis.

There is general agreement that surgery is the preferred treatment for adenoid cystic carcinoma.[63] Complete excision at the first surgical procedure has been shown to offer the patient the best chance for long-term survival and cure[10]. Elective regional lymph node dissection is not indicated, because distant metastasis is more common than cervical (regional) node involvement. With submandibular gland tumors, however, some type of node dissection is performed, since this conforms to established principles of surgery. Although complete surgical removal is a necessity relative to any chance for cure, Matsuba and colleagues have cautioned against extremely radical or mutilating surgery, particularly in the presence of distant metastasis.[64] According to Adam Maciejewski et al, radical surgical excision with margins proven to be histologically free of tumor with postoperative radiotherapy for all cases should be the treatment of choice. Lymph node dissection is recommended only in cases of histologically proven positive lymph nodes.[65] A frozen section diagnosis to achieve tumor free safe margins is necessary to specifically look for safe perineural margins because ACC is known to spread quickly along the nerve.

Conley J and Dingman DL, in 1974, have reported that adenoid cystic carcinoma is a radiosensitive tumor, and radiation therapy does play a role in the management of this disease, particularly in the control of microscopic disease after initial surgery or in treating local recurrent disease. They have also recommended radiation therapy for palliation of unresectable disease.[2] In cases of adenoid cystic carcinoma of the parotid gland, local control and preservation of function if possible, is the treatment of choice.[66] However, according to Conley, 1975, sacrifice of facial nerve becomes necessary to increase long-term local tumor control.[2]

In a study by Witten et al, local recurrences have been seen in almost 32% of the cases.[66] The risk of distant metastasis is also high, approximately 40%, and can occur in less than 8 years after treatment. This wide range of time in which local recurrences occur suggests that adenoid cystic carcinoma of the head and neck is a heterogenous group of tumors with the same histological feature.[57]

Acinic cell adenocarcinoma

Nasse, in 1892, described four parotid adenomas composed of cells that closely resembled the normal acinar cells. For the first half of the twentieth century, these acinar cell-like tumors were believed to be benign, and such terms as glandular epitheliomas, adenoma, salivary adenoma, parotid adenoma, and serous cell adenoma were applied. In 1953, Buxton and colleagues were the first to ascribe a malignant potential to many of these tumors, which they designated as serous cell adenocarcinomas. Later, Foote and Frazell and Godwin and coworkers reported series of parotid gland tumors that they classified as acinic cell adenocarcinomas.

Clinical features

The parotid gland is the predominant site of occurrence (83%), 3.8 percent in the submandibular gland, and 13 percent in the minor salivary glands according to the AFIP salivary gland registry. The buccal mucosa, upper lip, and palate, in that order, are the most frequent minor salivary gland sites of occurrence. The sublingual gland is a rare site of occurrence.[67] Acinic cell adenocarcinomas account for about 30 percent of all primary malignancies in the parotid gland, but only 7 percent of submandibular gland, 6 percent of sublingual gland, and 8 percent of minor gland malignant neoplasms. In the parotid gland, acinic cell adenocarcinoma is just behind mucoepidermoid carcinoma (33%) as the most frequently encountered salivary gland malignant tumor[67] In a study by Yih et al, 2005, acinic cell adenocarcinoma constituted only 0.5% of all tumors of the minor salivary glands.[68] Spiro et al, 1975, have reported an incidence of 12%.[69]

A female predominance has been observed by many. It was found to be 59% in the AFIP registry. The incidence among adult patients is evenly spread throughout the decades of life. The AFIP registry has recorded patients ranging from 3 to 91 years, the mean age being 44 years. Patients under 20 years made up 12.5 percent of the total patients.[67]

Acinic cell adenocarcinomas are usually slow growing al-though occasional tumors may have a more rapid enlargement. Symptoms include a long standing non tender, palpable mass. Patients have typically been aware of their tumor masses for less than a year, but some patients have reported being aware of the presence of the lesion for up to 30 years. Although they are considered low grade, they frequently recur locally or in the regional lymph nodes or in distant sites. Swelling, the principal symptom, is noted in nearly all cases; however, pain or tenderness is also experienced rather frequently. Facial nerve paralysis is infre-quent but is an ominous prognostic sign.[67]

Gross pathology[67]

Gross examination of parotidectomy specimens demonstrates acinic cell adenocarcinomas to be mononodular, well circumscribed, and 2 to 4 cm in diameter. However, multinodularity is not infrequent. Some tumors may appear to be encapsulated. In tissue sections, they are grayish white to reddish gray and lack the slimy texture of myxoid-type mixed tumors. They vary in consistency from firm to soft, may be somewhat friable, and may be solid or cystic. The cystic tumors usually have numerous small to microscopic cystic spaces, but larger cysts are occasionally present and may dominate the lesion.

The morphologic growth patterns can be described as solid, microcystic, papillary-cystic, and follicular. The individual cell characteristics can be categorized as acinar, intercalated duct like, vacuolated, clear, and nonspecific glandular. Any and all of these morphologic patterns and cell types may be seen in any specific tumor. In fact, 45 percent of these neoplasms manifest more than one growth pattern, and it is unusual for a tumor to be composed of only one cell type.

Histopathologic features[67]

On gross examination, many of these tumors are well circumscribed, but microscopic examination demonstrates that most are infiltrative. Acinar cell is the basis for the designation of these tumors as acinic cell adenocarcinomas.

These cells are usually readily identified by their relatively large size, round to polygonal shape, basophilic to amphophilic cytoplasm, and dark-staining cytoplasmic granules that are similar to those of normal parenchymal acinar cells. The amount of cytoplasmic granules varies from a few to many. The nuclei are round, eccentrically located, darkly stained, and very uniform from cell-to-cell. Periodic acid-Schiff stain highlights the cytoplasmic granules. The acinar cell is the predominant cell type observed in about 43 percent of the tumors, but some of these cells can be found in nearly all acinic cell adenocarcinomas.

The intercalated duct-like cells are smaller than acinar cells and cuboidal. Their cytoplasm is amphophilic to acidophilic. The nuclei are centrally placed and about the same size as the acinar cells; thus, the ratio of nuclei to cytoplasm is increased. The nuclei also appear hyperchromatic like the acinar cell nuclei. Often, these cells surround small lumina. Intercalated duct cells are the predominant cell type in approximately 32 percent of these neoplasms but can be seen in a very high percentage of cases. The vacuolated cells, about the size of the well-differentiated acinar cells, are unique to acinic cell adenocarcinomas among salivary gland neoplasms. However, some may appear to be distended due to presence of cytoplasmic vacuolae. They have eccentric nuclei that are less chromatic and more pleomorphic than those of acinar or intercalated duct-like cells. If evident, the cytoplasm is amphophilic to eosinophilic. However, the cytoplasmic compartment is punctuated by clear vacuoles that occupy most of the cytoplasm. Several vacuoles or a single large vacuole may be present. Stains for lipids and glycogen demonstrate no material in the vacuoles, but there may be some mucopolysaccharides. The vacuolated cells are most evident in the microcystic and papillary cystic growth patterns, where it appears that many of the cystic spaces may form by rupture of the, cell membranes

150 Salivary gland pathologies

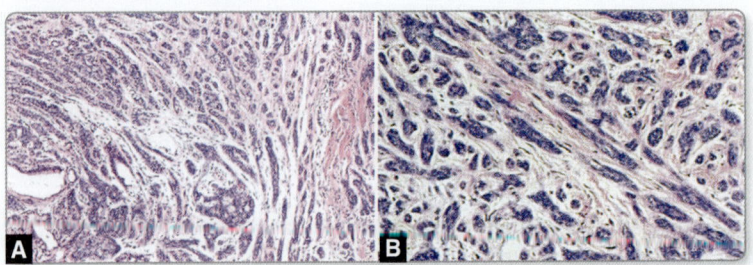

Figures 11.20A and B Photomicrograph of (A) Polymorphous low grade adenocarcinoma; (B) Under high magnification (40X)
(*Source:* Ellis GL, Editor. Surgical pathology of the salivary glands)

and coalescence of the vacuoles. Although the vacuolated cells are the predominant cell type in fewer than 10 percent of tumors, they are seen in about one-third of the neoplasms.

The nonspecific glandular cells form a syncytium of cells with indistinct cell boundaries and amphophilic cytoplasm. The nuclei are typically larger and more vesicular and pleomorphic than those of the other cell types. Although mitotic figures are infrequent in acinic cell adenocarcinomas, they are most evident in the nonspecific glandular cells.

A solid growth pattern is the most easily recognized morphologic variant of acinic cell adenocarcinoma because it usually contains large numbers of well-differentiated acinar cells and most closely resembles the normal parotid gland parenchyma. Groups of the tumor's acinar cells are separated and surrounded by very thin fibrous septa that contain small, nearly invisible capillaries. Clear cells often grow in solid sheets but are not the dominant cell type. Due to occasional presence of a capsule around the tumor, previously this tumor has been interpreted as benign. 38% of the tumors display a solid variety.

The microcystic pattern is extensive in one-third of acinic cell adenocarcinomas and can be found to a lesser extent in nearly another one third of these neoplasms. The microcystic pattern has numerous small cystic spaces, most of which are about three to ten times the size of acinar cells. Well-differentiated acinar cells are quite frequent and may even be the dominant cell type in this pattern; however, vacuolated and intercalated duct-like cells can also be prominent. Microcystic spaces may result from the coalescence of intracellular vacuoles of ruptured cells. Proteinaceous or mucinous material may pool in the microcystic spaces, but papillary projections of tumor cells into the cysts are absent.

The papillary-cystic growth pattern is characterized by one or more cystic structures that contain proliferations of epithelium. The cysts may be small with a few folds of lining epithelium projecting into the lumina. Other cystic structures can be quite large with long stalks, fronds, or masses of glandular epithelium within the lumina. Some of the epithelial projections have thin fibrovascular cores, whereas others appear to be masses of epithelium without apparent supporting stroma. These epithelial proliferations can vary in thickness from just a few cells to many cells and may assume a cystic or microcystic appearance of their own. Intercalated duct-like and nonspecific glandular cells usually predominate; however, vacuolated cells are often numerous, and acinar cells can be seen but well-differentiated acinar cells are frequently not conspicuous. The apical portions of many of the lumen-lining cells bulge into the lumen and produce a tombstone or hobnail-like conformation. Occasionally, these tumors present as single cysts that are lined by cuboidal epithelium with scattered papillary projections. In these cases, the tumors give the impression that they may have arisen from the epithelial lining of parotid cysts. The papillary--cystic pattern occurs less frequently than the microcystic or solid growth pattern.

The follicular pattern of acinic cell adenocarcinoma is the least frequently encountered. It is observed in only 10 percent of acinic cell adenocarcinomas, and it is the dominant pattern in only about one half of those. This pattern has a definite thyroid-like appearance. Variable-sized, ovoid to round cystic spaces are lined by cuboidal to low columnar epithelial cells. Many of the cystic spaces contain an eosinophilic proteinaceous material that simulates the appearance of colloid. The intercystic areas are usually occupied by epithelial cells that are mostly nonspecific glandular cells with some vacuolated and acinic type cells.

Acinic cell adenocarcinomas are frequently associated with a lymphoid infiltrate in the supporting stroma. This infiltrate is not just a scattering of inflammatory cells but a dense collection of lymphocytes in which even germinal centers may be evident. Prominent vascularity and hemorrhage may be associated with some of the collagenous regions. Psammoma-type calcifications, similar to those seen in thyroid papillary carcinoma, are occasionally found.

Some investigators have suggested segregating acinic cell adenocarcinomas into low-grade and high-grade neoplasms. In 1979, Batsakis and coworkers defined high-grade acinic cell adeno-carcinomas as having infiltrative growth; a medullary pattern, ductulotubular architecture, and prominence of undifferentiated cells. Their low-grade carcinomas manifested acinolobular, microcystic, and papillary growth patterns and were composed of, cells that had no ductuloglandular or tubular elements. However the authors commented that the grading system was fallible as occasionally patient with a low-grade carcinoma followed the same postoperative course as a patient with a high-grade carcinoma.

Management of acinic cell adenocarcinoma

Acinic cell adenocarcinomas are regarded as low-grade malignancies. If the tumor is confined to the superficial lobe of the parotid gland, at least superficial lobe parotidectomy is to be performed. When the deep lobe is involved, total parotidectomy is necessary. Local enucleation is to be avoided. If the facial nerve is uninvolved by tumor, preservation of the facial nerve is desirable. When the submandibular gland is the site of occurrence, complete resection of the gland is necessary. In the minor salivary glands, ensured complete local excision is needed. Radical neck dissection is not to be performed routinely but is used when there is clinical evidence of cervical lymph node involvement. Radiation as the only therapy is not recommended. Tu and colleagues have stated that postoperative radiation therapy does not increase the survival for patients with low-grade malignant parotid tumors, but in cases where there is doubt about the completeness of removal, and further surgery is not feasible because of extensive local disease, postoperative radiotherapy may be advantageous. Although acinic cell adenocarcinomas occur in the minor salivary glands infrequently, the prognosis for the minor gland tumors has been better than for those in the parotid gland.

According to Spiro et al, 1978, there was a recurrence rate of about 35 percent, a metastatic rate of 16 percent, and a death rate as a result of disease of 16 percent.[70]

Hickman and colleagues found the 5-year and 10-year survival rates for acinic cell adenocarcinoma to be 82 and 68 percent, respectively. In their series, which also included mucoepidermoid carcinoma, adenoid cystic carcinoma, mixed malignant tumor, this was the best tumor type.[71]

It has been shown in a study that about one half of the tumors that have recurred or metastasized have been well circumscribed without substantial infiltrative growth. On the other hand, multinodularity and stromal hyalinization have evinced in 70 and 60 percent, respectively, of acinic cell adenocarcinomas that recurred or metastasized. The clinical stage of the disease seems to be a more important prognostic factor than histopathologic features.[72]

Malignant mixed tumor

Malignant mixed tumors of salivary gland origin are relatively uncommon neoplasms. They include three different clinical and pathologic entities:
1. Carcinoma ex-mixed tumor (carcinoma arising in a mixed tumor),
2. Carcinosarcoma (true malignant mixed tumor), and
3. Metastasizing mixed tumor.

The first accounts for the vast majority of malignant mixed tumors, whereas the last two are extremely uncommon and account for only a small percentage of tumors in this group.

Carcinoma ex-mixed tumor

Carcinoma ex-mixed tumor is also known as carcinoma ex-pleomorphic adenoma or carcinoma arising in a mixed tumor. It is a mixed tumor in which a second neoplasm develops from the epithelial component that fulfills the criteria for malignancy.[73] These criteria includes invasiveness, destruction of normal tissues, cellular anaplasia, cellular pleomorphism, atypical mitoses, and abnormal architectural patterns, such as back-to-back glands and sheets of cells. Necrosis and increased numbers of normal-appearing mitotic figures should not be considered as indicative or diagnostic of malignancy. They occasionally have focal areas of marked epithelial atypia. Therefore, cellular atypia alone is insufficient for making a definitive diagnosis of malignancy and must be combined with other criteria before malignancy can be firmly established. When carcinoma ex-mixed tumor metastasizes, only the carcinoma component metastasizes; the benign mixed tumor component is not found in the metastases.

Clinical features

According to the Armed Forces Institute of Pathology (AFIP) registry, carcinoma ex-mixed tumors account for 2.2 percent of all types of tumors, 4.5 percent of all mixed tumors (benign and malignant combined), and 6.5 percent of all malignant tumors.[1] The mean ages for men and women were equivalent. Similar mean ages have been recorded by other authors however, Gerughty et al recorded a younger average age of 40 years. There is a lower incidence in children.[73] There is a slight predominance of female patients, with 55 percent of tumors occurring in women.

Eighty percent of the tumors, according to AFIP registry arose in the major salivary glands and 17.5 percent in the minor glands. Of those, 81 percent involved the parotid gland, 16.5 percent the submandibular gland, and 0.4 percent the sublingual gland. In the minor glands, 63 percent of tumors involved the palate; 10.5 percent the upper lip; 7 percent each the tongue, cheek, and oropharyngeal regions; and 5 percent other minor gland sites.

Most frequent symptom is a painless mass of long duration. In few of the cases there is history of sudden rapid growth and occasionally ulceration may be present. Pain may be manifested in a few cases. Pain is associated mainly with submandibular gland tumors. Presence of nerve palsy (38%) and fixation of tumor to the underlying structures (65%) is also seen in few cases.[74] The average size of carcinoma ex-mixed tumor is more than twice that of its benign counterpart, ranging from 1.5 to 25.0 cm in greatest dimension.[75]

Salivary gland pathologies

Histopathology[73]

Grossly, carcinoma ex-mixed tumor is usually poorly circumscribed, and many are extensively infiltrative. Occasional tumors, especially in the major glands, may be well circumscribed or completely encapsulated. The tumors have been described as hard and white or tangray.[76] The malignant areas in carcinoma ex-mixed tumor consist of epithelial cells with an increased nuclear cytoplasmic ratio, prominent nucleoli, and prominent numbers of mitoses. The most common histologic pattern in these areas is poorly differentiated adenocarcinoma or undifferentiated carcinoma, but tumors with epidermoid carcinoma, mucoepidermoid carcinoma, myoepithelial carcinoma, adenoid cystic carcinoma, clear cell carcinoma, papillary carcinoma and terminal duct carcinoma (polymorphous low-grade adenocarcinoma) also occur.

Destructive infiltrative growth is the most reliable histologic criterion for the diagnosis of a carcinoma ex-mixed tumor. Gerughty and colleagues suggested that histologic evidence of an invasive growth pattern, neural or vascular invasion, necrosis, and focal calcification implied a poor prognosis. The number of patients with neural involvement has varied among different series from a small percentage of tumors up to 55 percent of tumors.[77] Vascular invasion is observed somewhat less frequently, with up to 19 percent of tumors demonstrating vascular invasion. Mitotic figures are usually common, and in some studies, all tumors contain mitotic figures.

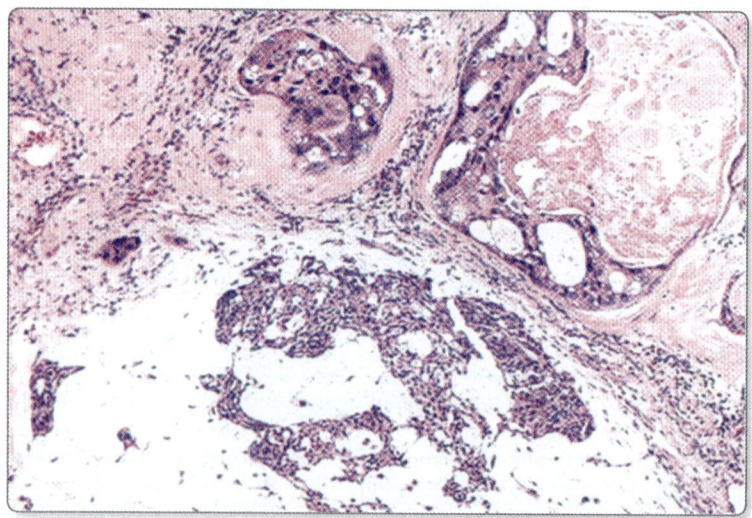

Figure 11. 21 Photomicrograph of carcinoma ex-pleomorphic adenoma (10X)
(*Source:* Ellis GL, Editor. Surgical pathology of the salivary glands)

Mitoses are much more commonly found in carcinoma ex-mixed tumors than in benign mixed tumors, In addition, there seems to be a positive correlation between the increasing frequency of occurrence of mitotic figures and more invasive growth patterns.[76] Carcinoma ex-mixed tumor seems to arise in two different situations: in primary or in recurrent mixed tumor. Eneroth and Zetterberg have suggested that as mixed tumors age, a population of cells may undergo transformation that could give origin to the carcinomatous component of carcinoma ex-mixed tumor. Many carcinomas ex-mixed tumors may have only small areas of residual mixed tumor. Therefore, a thorough examination of a carcinoma may be necessary to find these small foci for proper histologic classification.[73]

Management of carcinoma ex-mixed tumor

The best form of therapy seems to be wide surgical excision with a contiguous lymph node dissection and adjuvant radiation therapy. The adjuvant role of chemotherapy needs to be further evaluated; however, because of the high rate of distant metastasis with these tumors, it would appear to offer the potential of increased survival as better protocols become available. Radiotherapy as the only means of therapy has not proved effective. Carcinoma ex-mixed tumor is an aggressive tumor. Approximately 40 to 50 percent of patients develop one or more recurrences.[74,75,77] Tumors that arise in the submandibular gland or palate appear to have higher recurrence rate, that range to just over 70 percent, as cited by Spiro[77] whereas LiVolsi et al have demonstrated a lower recurrence rate for palatal tumors (12 percent)[77]. Nearly all the researchers have shown that prognosis in tumor recurrence is extremely poor and leads to death in most of the cases.

According to Gerughty, 1969, the metastatic rate varies from series to series, with up to 71 percent of patients developing local or distant metastases. Sites of distant metastases, in order of frequency, were lung, bone (especially the spine), abdominal viscera, and central nervous system.[73]

Tumors with the carcinomatous component contained within the tumor capsule have an excellent prognosis that is similar to that for benign mixed tumor.[77] Tumors penetrating the capsule have a poor prognosis, with 5-year survival rates in the range of 25 to 65 percent, 10-year survival rates of approximately 24 to 50 percent, 15-year survival rates of 10 to 35 percent.[74,78]

Tortoledo and colleagues found that no patients with invasion less than 8 mm from the capsule died from their tumor, whereas all patients with invasion greater than 9 mm beyond the capsule died secondary to their tumor. They also examined recurrence rates and the distance of invasion into adjacent tissues, and they found the local recurrence rates to be 70.5 percent when invasion exceeded 6 mm and 16.6 percent when invasion was less than 6 mm.[75]

Carcinosarcoma

Carcinosarcoma, also known as true malignant mixed tumor, is a tumor in which both the stromal and epithelial components fulfill histologic criteria of malignancy.[73] When these tumors metastasize, both components almost always, with rare exceptions, metastasize together.

Clinical features

Carcinosarcoma are rare tumors. The average incidence in published series is 0.4 percent (range 0.1–0.6 percent) of major salivary gland tumors and 1.0 percent (range 0.1–2.6 percent) of malignant salivary gland tumors.[73] The average age of patients at diagnosis for the eight cases at AFIP was 56.5 years (range 14 to 87 years).

The mean age of occurrence of this tumor as recorded in literature is 58.5 years with a range of 25 to 85 years. The frequency of occurrence is parotid followed by submandibular gland, and then minor glands in palate and tongue. This tumor might arise in a patient with a previously excised benign mixed tumor, or recurring benign mixed tumor or a locally metastasizing mixed tumor.

Tumors have ranged in size from 2 to 9 cm in maximum dimension.[7] Most common presenting symptom is an enlarging mass or a mass with a recent increase in size. Pain and/or facial paralysis may also occur. Rarely, patients present with metastases or experience difficulty swallowing or breathing. A patient with a central nervous system metastasis has been reported to present with headaches. The duration of symptoms before diagnosis ranged from 8 months to 40 years.[73]

Gross pathology[73]

The cut surface of the tumors is usually grayish in color, with rare yellowish regions and occasional areas with cystic change, hemorrhage, or calcification.

Histopathology[73]

The majority of carcinosarcomas are grossly infiltrative with poorly defined margins; occasional tumors are partially or totally encapsulated. Each of the tumors is biphasic with varying proportions and types of sarcomatous and carcinomatous elements. Sarcoma is the dominant tissue in the majority of tumors, with chondrosarcoma dominating the majority of specimens. Tumors may manifest areas of osteosarcoma, fibrosarcoma, high-grade sarcoma and malignant fibrous histiocytoma. Nonmalignant osteoid has also been rarely observed.[79] The carcinoma component of these tumors is most often a high-grade ductal adenocarcinoma or an undifferentiated carcinoma. Areas of epidermoid carcinoma are also observed, and regions with myoepithelial characteristics may be seen focally.

Management of carcinosarcoma

The data available is insufficient to recommend one type of therapy as definitive. However radical surgical excision, together with radiation therapy and lymph node dissection for palpable disease, seems to be the most prudent form of therapy.[73] The adjuvant role of chemotherapy needs to be further evaluated. Because of the high rate of distant metastasis with these tumors, it would appear to offer the potential for increased survival as better protocols become available. Radiotherapy as the only means of therapy has not proved effective.

There is a mean length of survival of 29.3 months, according to literature. Patients die from locally recurrent and/or metastatic disease. Fourteen tumors (54%) metastasized either locally or to distant sites. Tumors metastasized more than twice as often to the lung than to any other single anatomic site. Hilar and cervical lymph nodes were the next most frequent sites; however, distant metastases were also rarely found in various soft tissue sites, bone, liver, and in the central nervous system.

Metastasizing mixed tumor

Metastasizing mixed tumor is a salivary gland tumor that is histologically identical to benign mixed tumor, with both the epithelial and stromal components having a benign appearance. Yet, for some unknown reason, the tumor metastasizes. The metastases in this tumor contain both the epithelial and stromal components found in typical mixed tumors. Earlier literature has referred to these tumors as "benign" metastasizing mixed tumors but because they may be lethal, they are now referred to as metastasizing mixed tumor and the adjective "benign" is no more used.

Clinical features[73]

It is a very rarely experienced tumor. According to literature, there is no particular sex predilection. It chiefly occurs in the parotid gland. Most of the patients have a history surgical excision of a benign mixed tumor.

Clinically, patients initially present with painless masses similar to typical benign mixed tumors. Metastatic lesions are often found on chest radiographs or produce symptoms relative to the location of the metastases, such as back pain for spinal metastases, painless neck masses for cervical lymph node metastases, and epigastric discomfort for a liver metastasis.

Histopathology[73]

Both primary and metastatic tumors have a cellular composition typical of the range of benign mixed tumor of salivary gland origin which has already been discussed. Both epithelial and stromal-like components are usually found, although a rare metastasis may contain only myoepithelial cells.

Necrosis and prominent mitotic activity are lacking, although occasional tumors demonstrate epithelial atypia. Characteristics of malignancy are always lacking. Several primary tumors have had a predominant mucoid appearance. In benign mixed tumors, this histologic pattern has been associated with a higher recurrence rate, and it has been postulated by El-Naggar and colleagues that repeated surgical manipulation may allow possible access of tumor cells to vascular spaces. However, vascular invasion has yet to be demonstrated in any metastasizing mixed tumor, although several cases of typical benign mixed tumor with vascular invasion within the tumor proper have been reported by Thomas et al, 1980.[80]

Previous surgical manipulation may be a necessary factor for the mixed tumor to metastasize, since in all cases reported patients have undergone surgical excision prior to the diagnosis of Metastasizing mixed tumor. Therefore, surgical manipulation in combination with other factors yet to be determined, such as vascular invasion and tumor embolization, is the most likely explanation for tumor metastases.

Management of metastasizing mixed tumor

The best form of therapy appears to be wide local excision for both the primary and metastatic tumors. The role of radiation therapy and/or chemotherapy is still under evaluation.

The tumor has a poor prognosis because of the distant metastasis that does occur to vital organs. Half of these tumors metastasize to bone (including the middle to lower spine, iliac region, rib, skull, mandible, femur, and humerus), 30 percent metastasize to the lung and 30 percent to the lymph nodes, usually in the lymphatic drainage region of the primary tumor. Less common sites of spread included the scalp, the abdominal wall, and the liver.

Primary squamous cell carcinoma

Primary squamous cell carcinomas are unique among salivary gland tumors in several respects. Their frequency of occurrence and morphologic appearance are similar to that of squamous cell carcinomas that metastasize to or secondarily involve the glands. The diagnosis of primary squamous cell carcinoma is limited to the major glands because distinction between possible minor salivary gland primary tumors and those originating from mu-cosal surface epithelium is generally not possible.

Clinical features[81]

According to AFIP registry, the mean age of occurrence of this malignancy is 60.5 years, the range being 7.0 to 95.0 years. Male predilection for occurrence of this tumor is noticed at a ratio of 2:1 in AFIP registry; whereas

Shemen LJ et al have noticed a near equal incidence. The predilection for occurrence of this tumor is in the parotid gland followed by submandibular and sublingual gland.[82]

The most common presenting symptom of patients with parotid tumors is an asymptomatic mass. Nonetheless, patients may also present with pain and facial nerve palsy. The size of the masses might vary, but is usually greater than 3 cm. Submandibular squamous cell carcinoma often replaces the entire gland and may be manifested as a painful mass. Occasionally patients are asymptomatic. Fixation to skin and/or deep structures is also encountered.

In a study by Shemen et al, symptoms were present for less than 1 year in about 75 percent of the patients and rarely were present for more than 2 years.[82]

Gross pathology[81]

On gross examination, these tumors appear unencapsulated, and the tumor interface is often difficult to distinguish from the salivary gland parenchyma. As with other squamous cell carcinomas, these tumors are firm or hard, and the cut surface is light gray or white. Occasionally, extensive parenchymal invasion is accompanied by extension of tumor into the dermis overlying the gland which suggests possible epidermal origin.

Histopathology[81]

Histologically, these tumors are similar to squamous cell carcinomas from other sites. Since cytoplasmic mucin is not found in this tumor, special stains for mucus should be routinely performed to ensure that the tumor is not a high-grade mucoepidermoid carcinoma.

Most tumors are well or moderately differentiated keratinizing squamous cell carcinomas. Trabeculae of desmoplastic fibrous connective tissue often separate the tumor into multiple nodules. Few might originate in dysplastic salivary ducts. Squamous cell carcinomas often overrun the glandular parenchyma, which leaves small remnants of metaplastic ducts or degenerating acini surrounded by desmoplastic fibrous tissue. Desmoplasia may be so pronounced that entire salivary gland lobules are replaced by fibrous connective tissue that contains scattered tumor islands. Intracellular keratin and keratin pearl formation are normally prominent, and intercellular bridges are evident.

Differential diagnosis[81]

Ductal squamous metaplasia, high-grade mucoepidermoid carcinoma, lymphoepithelial carcinoma should be considered in the differential diagnosis of squamous cell carcinoma of the salivary gland.

Management and prognosis

The management is chiefly surgical. Patients with parotid tumors are treated with parotidectomy with or without preservation of the facial nerve as per the merit of the case. In case of submandibular gland tumor, the entire gland is resected. With tumors from either gland, a concurrent neck dissection is performed if cervical metastases are clinically evident or suspected. Because locoregional failure is overall the most significant problem, it is suggested that a composite resection might be appropriate for most sizeable tumors that involve the capsule of the submandibular gland. Postoperative radiotherapy when combined with surgery, may improve locoregional control.[83] A study by Shemen and coworkers indicated that the presence of ulceration or fixation, advanced patient age, and advanced tumor stage contributed to a poor prognosis. Histologic grade does not influence survival.[82]

Clear cell carcinoma

Clear cell neoplasms of salivary glands have been classified as both adenomas and carcinomas. The terminology employed for these neoplasms includes adenomyoepithelioma, clear cell adenoma, glycogen-rich adenoma, glycogen-rich carcinoma or adenocarcinoma, clear cell carcinoma, glycogen-rich tumor, clear cell tumor, monomorphic clear cell tumor, and epithelial-myoepithelial carcinoma.[84]

Clinical features[84]

It is encountered in the minor salivary glands in approximately 57% of the cases with palate being the most dominant site whereas in parotid and submandibular glands, incidence is 28 and 12% respectively. There is no sex or racial predilection. It occurs at age range of 18 to 86 years, mean age being 56 years. Clinically it is manifested as a swelling like other salivary gland tumors.

Gross pathology[84]

These tumors appear to be circumscribed on gross examination, but usually are not encapsulated. The cut surfaces are grayish-white to grayish tan.

Histopathology[84]

Most dominant feature of this tumor is tumor cells with cytoplasm that do not stain with hematoxylin and eosin. Although clear cells are the most conspicuous feature, a number of cells, can be found with pale eosinophilic

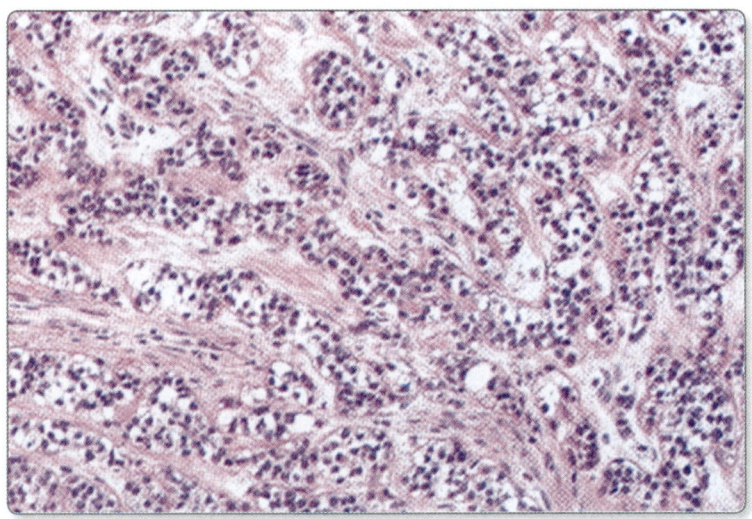

Figure 11. 22 Photomicrograph of clear cell carcinoma (10X)
(*Source:* Ellis GL, Editor. Surgical pathology of the salivary glands)

or amphophilic cytoplasm. The tumor cells are round to polygonal and vary in size. The nuclei are generally fairly uniform with little pleomorphism and few or no mitotic figures. The chromatin is evenly dispersed, and nucleoli are not prominent. At least some glycogen is seen in most clear cell carcinomas. Clear cell carcinomas manifest several growth patterns. The tumors may grow as solid sheets, small nests, or cords of epithelial cells.

Infiltration is characteristic. When these tumors develop as small nests or cords in an extensive fibrous stroma, they are usually easily recognized as carcinomas because of their obvious infiltrative appearance. When these tumors are composed of large sheets of cells and occur in the major salivary glands, a condensation of fibrous tissue frequently occurs at the tumor periphery and imparts an encapsulated appearance leading to a mistaken diagnosis of clear cell "adenomas."

Differential diagnosis[84]

Diagnosis may be confused with mucoepidermoid carcinoma and acinic cell adenocarcinoma which are two common malignant salivary gland tumors that may occasionally contain a significant number of clear cells. Metastatic renal cell carcinoma must always be considered in the differential diagnosis of clear cell tumors. A positive reaction to mucicarmine would preclude the possibility of renal cell carcinoma.

Management and prognosis

All clear cell tumors, apart from the rare clear cell oncocytoma, should be regarded as at least potentially malignant and treated accordingly due to their infiltrative growth and the incidence of recurrence and of regional lymph node metastases, it is appropriate to consider them low-grade adenocarcinomas. Consistent with their low-grade malignant status, partial or complete parotidectomy or sublingual glandectomy, complete submandibular glandectomy, and wide local excision of minor gland tumors are recommended forms of treatment.

Epithelial–myoepithelial carcinoma

The epithelial-myoepithelial carcinoma of intercalated duct origin is a rare biphasic type of low-grade salivary gland carcinoma that constitutes less than 1 percent of salivary gland neoplasms.

Clinical features[85]

Epithelial-myoepithelial carcinoma is most prevalent in older individuals, with approximately two thirds of the tumors occurring in the sixth and seventh decades of life. The neoplasm exhibits a predilection for female patients. Epithelial-myoepithelial carcinoma may arise in any salivary tissue, but it has a predilection for the parotid gland. Clinically, most patients present with an asymptomatic or painful salivary gland swelling with a history of steady increase in size over an extended period of time.[86] Patients may also complain of facial paralysis.[87] Nasal obstruction and facial deformity may represent major complaints of patients with maxillary involvement.[88]

Gross pathology[85]

They occur as single, well-circumscribed, firm, lobulated, neoplasms that usually range in size from 2 to 8 cm. They are typically bosselated neoplasms and on cross-sectional examination exhibit a multinodular growth pattern with irregular cystic spaces. It is not unusual for these tumors to have an infiltrative growth pattern. In addition, recurrent tumors may exhibit superficial lobulation or multicentric growth with irregular tumor borders and central areas of necrosis.

Histopathology[85]

This tumor shows a multinodular growth pattern with islands of tumor cells separated by dense bands of fibrous connective tissue. The islands of tumor cells are composed of small ducts lined with cuboidal epithelium that is surrounded by clear cells that interface with a thickened, hyaline like

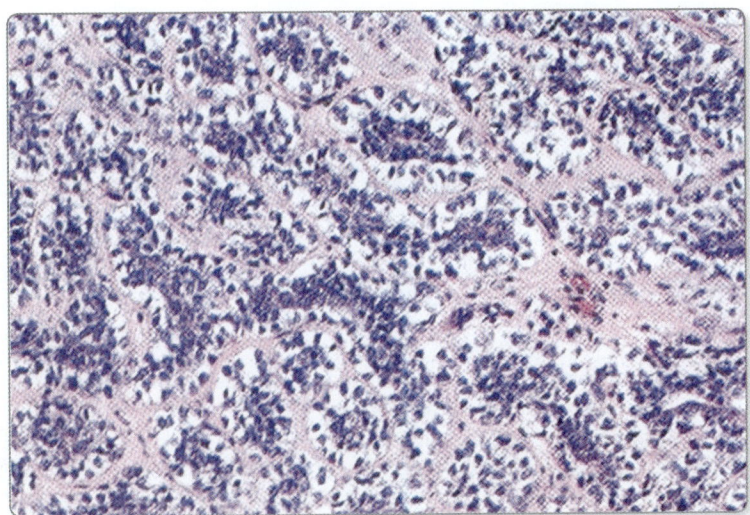

Figure 11.23 Photomicrograph of epithelial-myoepithelial carcinoma (10X) (*Source:* Ellis GL, Editor. Surgical pathology of the salivary glands)

basement membrane. The inner, luminal cuboidal cells have finely granular, dense, eosinophilic cytoplasm and central or basally located round nuclei.

Columnar cells and squamous foci may also be seen proliferating within cystic and micro cystic spaces that often contain material that reacts positively to periodic acid-Schiff (PAS) stain. The outer, clear myoepithelial cells vary in shape from columnar to ovoid and have well-defined cell borders and eccentrically located vesicular nuclei located toward the basement membrane. The tumors' growth patterns may vary from solid lobules that are separated by bands of hyalinized, vascular, fibrous connective tissue to irregular, papillary cystic arrangements with tumor cells that partially or completely fill cyst-like spaces. Generally, if a fibrous capsule is present, it is infiltrated by tumor cells, which results in satellitosis of the tumor element. The dense, hyaline, basement-membrane like material that separates islands of tumor cells stains strongly with PAS and periodic acid-methenamine silver stains.

Differential diagnosis[85]

The tumors to be considered for differential diagnosis include pleomorphic adenoma, acinic cell adenocarcinoma, adenoid cystic carcinoma, mucoepidermoid carcinoma, sebaceous carcinoma, and oncocytoma.

Management and prognosis

Surgery is considered the primary mode of treatment. Total parotidectomy is advocated for tumors in the parotid gland, and the facial nerve branches should be resected if they are involved by tumor.

Even with complete surgical resection, recurrences and distant metastasis remain a concern and may occur from a few months to years after the initial surgery.[89]

Undifferentiated carcinomas

This group includes three distinct entities:
1. Lymphoepithelial carcinomas (malignant lymphoepithelial lesion).
2. Undifferentiated large cell carcinomas.
3. Undifferentiated small cell carcinomas.

Lymphoepithelial carcinomas exhibit architectural features and histomorphologic growth patterns similar to those of the benign lymphoepithelial lesion. The small cell types bear a resemblance to oat cell carcinomas arising in other sites, whereas the large cell tumors resemble the undifferentiated carcinomas of the naso-pharynx.

Lymphoepithelial carcinoma

In 1962, Hilderman and others described an epithelial malignancy of the parotid gland resembling benign lymphoepithelial lesion. Since then, the malignant lymphoepithelial lesion has been recognized as a distinct entity with well-defined histopathologic features.[90] The term malignant lymphoepithelial lesion is confusing, as it fails to identify the malignant cell type (lymphoid or epithelial). Hence, the term lymphoepithelial carcinoma is preferred which clarifies that the epithelial component rather than the lymphoid element is malignant.

Clinical features[90]

Clinically, the overall female to male ratio for cases reported in the literature (regardless of ethnic background) is slightly less than 2 to 1. Gender predilections for these tumors vary according to race and ethnicity. Among Eskimos, a preponderance of female patients is notable, whereas lymphoepithelial carcinoma occurring among Chinese patients manifests a slight male predilection.[91]

According to Krisnamurthy et al, 1983, the mean age for patients with lymphoepithelial carcinoma at the time of diagnosis is 44 years for males and 36 years for females.[90]

The parotid gland is most commonly involved followed by submandibular gland. The average duration of signs or symptoms is 1.5

years. The primary physical finding is an indurated mass in the parotid region; pain or discomfort being a complaint among 50% of the patients, and drainage may be observed. Facial paralysis is observed in less than 20 percent of the patients.

Benign lymphoepithelial lesion preceding the emergence of lymphoepithelial carcinoma by many years has been reported, chiefly in whites, which is of clinical significance.[92]

Gross pathology[90]

The tumor is solid and measures 2 to 3 cm, although it could achieve a massive size. In the parotid gland, the tumor is firm and fixed yet usually circumscribed. Tumors have been variably described as grossly encapsulated, partially circumscribed, multinodular, and infiltrative. Cross-sections of tumor tissue vary from gray-tan to yellow-gray. Zonal necrosis and hemorrhage are rarely seen.

Histopathology[90]

At lower magnifications, lymphoepithelial carcinoma resembles benign lymphoepithelial lesion with oval and irregular elongated epithelial islands that occasionally anastomose and that are isolated by a benign lymphoid stroma. Acini and ducts may also be seen, particularly at the periphery, effaced by lymphoid infiltrates. Germinal centers and fibrosis may be evident.

At higher magnification, the epithelial cells appear polygonal to spindled, without keratinization or formation of lumina. The nuclei are large and somewhat vesicular. Mitoses are seen, but anaplasia is usually not a prominent finding. The epithelial element is solid, lacking any orientation around residual ducts. The lymphoid stroma includes plasma cells and immunoblasts as well as occasional epithelioid histiocytes, which may palisade about foci of fibrinous material, yielding a granulomatous appearance. The small lymphocytes are mature with regular nuclear membranes. Areas of fibrosis and hyalinization are common. In many cases, foci of neoplastic epithelial cells that are located in a fibrous stroma devoid of any prominent lymphoid infiltration may be present. Perineural invasion is frequently seen.

They may be graded as low – high grade based on histology. Lower grade lesion tends to resemble benign lymphoepithelial lesion more closely, with germinal centers and circumscription, but these lesions are more disorderly, with syncytial epithelium tending to form distinct trabeculae, sheets, and anastomosing islands. The cells tend to have vesicular nuclei with single nucleoli and easily recognized mitoses but no anaplasia. The neoplastic islands may envelop atypical acini and ducts; but true epimyoepithelial islands are not seen in the central regions of the tumor. A higher - grade lesion shows more diffuse infiltration of the epithelial islands by lymphoid cells, and germinal center formation is much less noticeable.

Differential diagnosis

The differential diagnosis of lymphoepithelial carcinoma includes squamous carcinoma and high-grade mucoepidermoid carcinoma in which a significant degree of lymphoid infiltration is present, poorly differentiated large cell carcinoma of salivary origin, and nasopharyngeal carcinoma with parotid extension or metastasis to lymph nodes of the parotid region.

Background lymphoid infiltrate and the typical architecture simulating benign lymphoepithelial lesion should help eliminate the first three lesions from consideration. A lack of any adenomatous features, particularly mucus-secreting cells, eliminates consideration of mucoepidermoid carcinoma. Papillary cystadenoma lymphomatosum that has undergone malignant transformation should also be considered. However, it is extremely rare and a characteristic morphology of Warthin's tumor is retained, while within the benign tumor mass a focus of adenocarcinoma is present.

Management and prognosis

Treatment for lymphoepithelial carcinoma consists of surgery alone or of surgery in combination with radiotherapy. Surgical therapy varies from local excision to radical excision with neck dissection.

Undifferentiated large cell carcinomas

Undifferentiated large cell carcinoma is defined as any tumor of salivary gland origin that exhibits a predominant poorly differentiated large cell component that occurs in islands or sheets, although minor foci within the tumor that exhibit some degree of adenoid or squamoid tendencies for differentiation may be present.[90]

Clinical features[90]

The tumor shows a predilection for occurrence in males. It occurs in an age range from 21 to 86 years with a mean age of 62.7 years. The undifferentiated large cell lesions affect an older population. It is seen most commonly in parotid gland followed by submandibular gland and minor salivary glands.

Gross pathology[90]

They lack encapsulation and are represented by grayish white infiltrative solid masses that are frequently found to extend into adjacent fascial and muscular tissues. Fixation to skin is commonly encountered, as is invasion of craniomaxillary osseous tissue and associated foramina. In tissue sections, the tumors are solid, cystic, and necrotic; hemorrhagic foci are unusual.

Histopathology[90]

According to Thackray and Lucas, undifferentiated carcinoma is a malignant tumor of epithelial structure that is too poorly differentiated to be placed in any of the other groups of carcinomas. Tubules, ductules, acinar structures, and keratin are not seen. However, if the malignancy arises out of pre-existing mixed tumor, adenoid cystic carcinoma, squamous cell carcinoma, or adenocarcinoma, morphologic remnants may be admixed.

The tumor cells are usually polygonal or spindled, and they infiltrate in sheets or as thin trabeculae or cords separated by fibrovascular stroma. Zonal necrosis and hemorrhage may be present along with a high mitotic rate.

Differential diagnosis

The differential diagnosis should include nasopharyngeal carcinoma with extension or metastasis to the parotid region, amelanotic melanoma, non-Hodgkin's lymphoma, lymphoepithelial carcinoma, olfactory neuroblastoma, and sarcomas, including rhabdomyosarcoma, synovial sarcoma, malignant epithelioid schwannoma, and malignant fibrous histiocytoma. A variety of metastatic large cell undifferentiated carcinomas must be ruled out as well.

Prognosis

Hui and colleagues, in their evaluation of both large and small cell lesions, observed that 53 percent of their subjects had recurrences, regional node metastases developed in 53 percent, distant metastases developed in 63 percent, and 63 percent died because of tumor. The most significant harbinger of a poor prognosis was found to be tumor size. Patients with lesions smaller than 4 cm had a mean survival time of 46 months, with 50 percent dying because of disease. When the tumors exceeded 4 cm, the mean patient survival time was 7.7 months, and 100 percent died from disease. Other indicators of poor prognosis were invasion of nerves larger than 0.25 mm and lymph node and distant metastases.[93]

Small cell carcinoma

Small cell carcinoma is a rare salivary gland tumor. It is a common pulmonary neoplasm, which rarely arises in the region of the head and neck. Most common site of involvement in the head neck region is the larynx but small cell carcinoma has also been reported to arise in the paranasal sinuses, oral cavity, nose, pharynx and cervical esophagus.

Undifferentiated carcinomas account for 0.3 to 3.2 percent of salivary gland tumors.[94]

Salivary gland pathologies

Clinical features[90]

Patients with small cell carcinomas of the major glands present most commonly during the fifth to seventh decades of life. There appears to be a slight male predominance, with 1.6 times as many tumors occurring in men than in women. 85% of the small cell carcinomas arise in the parotid gland, and the remainder involves the submandibular gland.

Patients present with non tender to painful masses, many of which are rapidly growing, measuring up to 8 cm in greatest dimension. The masses are usually present for less than 3 months; however, occasional patients have symptoms related to the tumor for periods of up to 1 year.

Gross pathology

Tumor margins are usually poorly demarcated with infiltrating edges; a rare tumor may be well circumscribed. Tumor consistency has been described as firm to hard, whereas color varies, including gray, gray-white, pink-gray to yellow-white, tan, and yellow.[95]

Histopathology[90]

The tumors are composed of infiltrating large sheets, ribbons, cords, or nests of anaplastic round-to-oval cells with minimal cytoplasm and hyperchromatic nuclei containing finely dispersed chromatin and inconspicuous nucleoli. Mitoses are frequent, and tumor necrosis is usually prominent. Vascular invasion, a common characteristic of small cell carcinomas at other sites, is only occasionally observed. Perineural invasion and rosette formation are occasionally found.

Differential diagnosis

The differential diagnosis of primary small cell carcinoma includes metastatic small cell carcinoma, undifferentiated large cell carcinoma of salivary gland origin, non-Hodgkin's lymphoma, poorly differentiated adenocarcinoma and epidermoid carcinoma, and solid adenoid cystic carcinoma. If tissue is well fixed and careful attention is paid to the small cell size, and if certain criteria are met, including lack of prominent nucleoli, minimal cytoplasm, fine chromatin distribution, prominent areas of necrosis, and a negative mucicarmine stain, most of the differential diagnostic possibilities should be eliminated.

Management and prognosis

The treatment of choice is wide surgical excision, possibly with radiation and/or chemotherapy. A lymphadenectomy should be reserved only for palpable disease, since this tumor tends to metastasize via a hematogenous route.

The prognosis for patients with small cell carcinomas arising in the major or minor salivary glands is better than that for patients with small cell carcinomas of the lung or larynx. 2-year and 5-year rates of survival for patients with small cell carcinomas arising in the major salivary glands were found to be 70 and 46 percent, respectively, whereas those for patients with small cell carcinoma of the larynx were 16 and 5 percent, respectively.[90,91,94] The most significant predictor of poor prognosis in this latter study was tumor size; patients with tumors less than 4 cm had a mean survival of 46 months, whereas those with tumors greater than 4 cm survived only 7.7 months, with 100 percent mortality. Other negative predictors of survival were nerve invasion and lymph node metastasis.

References

1. Spitz MR, Batsakis JG. Major salivary gland carcinoma. Arch Otolaryngol. 1984;110:45.
2. WHO manual of classification of diseases 2003.
3. Hanna EY, Suen JY. Malignant tumors of the salivary glands. Myers EN, Suen JY, Myers JN, Hanna EY, (Eds). Cancer of the head and neck, 4th edn. Saunders. 21:475-510.
4. Saunders JR, Hirata RM, Jaques DA. Salivary Glands. Surg clin of N Am. 1986; 66(1):59-81.
5. Johns M, Nachlas N. Salivary gland tumors Paperella, Shumrick, Gluckman, Meyerhoff editors. Otolaryngology. WB Saunders Company, Philafelphia, 3rd 1991;20(3):2099-127.
6. Ord RA. Surgical management of parotid tumors. Oral and Maxillofac Surg Clin of N Am1995;7(3):529-64.
7. Shafer W, Hine M, Levy B. Tumors of the salivary glands. A textbook of Oral Pathology. 4th edn. Harcourt Asia Pte. Ltd. 2000;3:230-57.
8. Cornog JL, Gray SR. Surgical and clinical pathology of salivary gland tumors. Rankow RM, Polayes IM, (Eds). Diseases of salivary glands. WB Saunders, Philadelphia 1976;5:99-142.
9. Johns M, Nachlas N. Salivary gland tumors. Paperella, Shumrick, Gluckman, Meyerhoff (Eds). Otolaryngology WB Saunders Company, Philadelphia. 1991;20(3)2099-127.
10. GR Seward. Nodular enlargement of a salivary gland. Moore, (Ed). Surgery of the Mouth and Jaws. Blackwell Scientific Publication, London. 1985;38:676-99.
11. Norman JE, McGurk M. History of salivary glands and mixed parotid tumor. Colour atlas and text of salivary glands-diseases, disorders and surgery. Mosby-Wolfe, Spain. 1995;1:1.
12. Waldron CA. Mixed tumor (Pleomorphic adenoma) and Myoepithelioma. Ellis GL, (Ed). Surgical pathology of the salivary glands. WB Saunders, Philadelphia. 1991;10:165-86.

13. Nayar R, Schindler S. Head and Neck. Haber MH, Gattuso P, Spitz DJ, David O (Eds). Differential diagnosis in surgical pathology, WB Saunders Co; Philadelphia. 2002;6:363-454.
14. Papadogeorgakis N, Skouteris CA, Mylonas AI, Angelopoulos AP. Superficial parotidectomy: technical modifications based on tumor characteristics. J Cranio Maxillofacs Surg. 2004;32:350-3.
15. von Glass W, Pesch HJ, Djauli R, Krause J. Surgery of pleomorphic adenoma of the parotid gland. HNO. 1989;37(10):426-31.
16. Grage TB, Morrow CE. Salivary gland neoplasms. McQuarrie DG, Adams GL, Shons AR, Browne GA, (Eds). Head and neck Cancer. Clinical decisions and management principles. Year book medical publishers Inc, Chicago, 20:369-86.
17. Warnock GR. Papillary Cystadenoma Lymphomatosum (Wharton's tumor. Ellis GL, (Ed). Surgical pathology of the salivary glands. WB Saunders, Philadelphia. 1991;11:187-201.
18. Cornog JL, Gray SR. Surgical and clinical pathology of salivary gland tumors. Rankow RM, Polayes IM, (Eds). Diseases of Salivary glands. WB Saunders, Philadelphia. 1976;5:99-142.
19. Batsakis JG. Tumors of the head and neck – Clinical and pathological considerations. Williams and Wilkins, Baltimore. 1979;1.
20. Eneroth CM. Salivary gland tumors in the parotid gland, submandibular gland and the palate region. Cancer. 1971;27:1415-8.
21. Saunders JR, Hirata RM, Jaques DA. Salivary Glands. Surg Clin of N Am. 1986; 66(1):59-81.
22. Ord RA. Surgical management of Parotid tumors. Oral and Maxillofac Surg Clin of N Am.1995;7(3):529-64.
23. GYYU, DQ Ma, XB Liu, MY Zhang, Q Zhang. Local excision of the parotid gland in the treatment of Warthin's tumor. Br J Oral Maxillofac Surg. 1988;36:186-9.
24. Goode RK. Oncocytoma. Ellis GL, (Ed). Surgical pathology of the salivary glands. WB Saunders, Philadelphia. 1991;13:225-37.
25. Shafer W, Hine M, Levy B. Tumors of the salivary glands. A textbook of Oral Pathology. 4th edn. Harcourt Asia Pte. Ltd. 2000;3:230-57.
26. Blank C, Eneroth CM, Jakobsson PA. Oncocytoma of the parotid gland: Neoplasm or nodular hyperplasia. Cancer. 1970;24:919-25.
27. Shafer W, Hine M, Levy B. Tumors of the salivary glands. A textbook of Oral Pathology. 4th edn; Harcourt Asia Pte. Ltd. 2000;3:230-57.
28. Kratochvil FJ. Canalicular adenoma and Basal cell adenoma. Ellis GL, Editor. Surgical pathology of the salivary glands. WB Saunders, Philadelphia 1991; 12:202-24.
29. Cornog JL, Gray SR. Surgical and clinical pathology of salivary gland tumors. Rankow RM, Polayes IM, Eds. Diseases of Salivary Glands. WB Saunders, Philadelphia. 1976;5:99-142.
30. Kratochvil FJ. Canalicular adenoma and Basal cell adenoma. Ellis GL, Editor. Surgical pathology of the salivary glands. WB Saunders, Philadelphia. 1991;12:202-24.

31. Waldron CA, El-Mofty SK, Gnepp DR. Tumors of the intraoral minor salivary glands: A demographic and histologic study of 426 cases. Oral Surg Oral Med Oral Pathol. 1988;66:323-33.
32. Christ TF, Crocker D. Basal cell adenoma of minor salivary gland origin. Cancer 1972;30:214-9.
33. Daley TD. The canalicular adenoma: Considerations on differential diagnosis and treatment. J Oral Maxillofac Surg. 1984;42:728-30.
34. Ellis GL, Auclair PL. Ductal papillomas. Ellis GL, (Ed). Surgical pathology of the salivary glands. WB Saunders, Philadelphia. 1991;14:238-51.
35. Regezi JA, Llyod RV, Zarbo RJ, McClatchey KD. Minor salivary gland tumors: A histologic and immunohistochemical study. Cancer. 1985;55:108-15.
36. Rennie JS, MacDonald DG, Critchlow HA. Sialadenoma papilliferum: A case report and review of the literature. Int J Oral Surg. 1984;13:452-4.
37. White DK, Miller AS, McDaniel RK, Rothman BN. Inverted ductal papilloma: A distinctive lesion of minor salivary gland. Cancer. 1982;49:519-24.
38. Kerpel SM, Freedman PD, Lumerman H. The papillary cystadenoma of minor salivary gland origin. Oral Surg Oral Med Oral Pathol 1978;46:820-6.
39. Bell RB, Dierks EJ, Homer L, Potter BE. Management and outcome of patients with malignant salivary gland tumors. J Oral Maxillofac Surg. 2005;63:917-28.
40. Plambeck K, Friedrich RE, Schmelzle R. Mucoepidermoid carcinoma of salivary gland origin: classification, clinical-pathological correlation, treatment results and long-term follow-up in 55 patients. Journal of Cranio-Maxillofacial Surgery 1996;24:133-9.
41. Auclair PL, Ellis GL. Mucoepidermoid carcinoma. Surgical Pathology of the salivary glands. WB Saunders, Philadelphia. 1991;16:269-98.
42. Castro EB, Huvos AG, Strong EW, Foote FW Jr. Tumors of major salivary glands in children, Cancer. 1972;29:312-7.
43. Healey WV, Perzin KH, Smith L. Mucoepidermoid carcinoma of salivary gland origin: Classification, clinical-pathologic correlation, and results of treatment. Cancer. 1970;26:368-88.
44. Neville BW, Damm DD, Weir JC, Fantasia JE. Labial salivary gland tumors, Cancer. 1988;61:2113-6.
45. Goldblatt LI, Ellis GL. Salivary gland tumors of the tongue. Analysis of 55 new cases and review of literature, Cancer. 1987;60:74-81.
46. Triantafillidou K, Dimitrakopoulos J, Iordanidis F, Koufogiannis D. Mucoepidermoid carcinoma of minor salivary glands: a clinical study of 16 cases and review of the literature. Oral Dis. 2006;12(4):364-70.
47. Olsen KD, Devine KD, Weiland LH. Mucoepidermoid carcinoma of the oral cavity. Otolaryngol Head Neck Surg. 1981;89:783-91.
48. Tran L, Sadeghi A, Hanson D, Ellerbroek N, Calcaterra TC, Parker RG. Salivary gland tumors of the palate: The UCLA experience. Laryngoscope. 1987;97:1343-45.
49. Vedrine PO, Coffinet L, Temam S, Montagne K, Lapeyre M, Oberlin O. Mucoepidermoid carcinoma of salivary glands in the pediatric age group: 18

clinical cases, including 11 second malignant neoplasms. Head Neck. 2006 Jun 16;in press.
50. Connell HC, Evans JC. Mucoepidermoid carcinoma of the salivary glands. Am J Surg.1972;124:519-21.
51. Tran L, Sadeghi A, Hanson D, Juillard G, Mackintosh R, Calcaterra TC, Parker RG. Major salivary gland tumors. Treatment results and prognostic factors. Laryngoscope 1986;96:1139-44.
52. Thorvaldsson SE, Beahrs OH, Woolner LB, Simons JH. Mucoepidermoid tumors of the major salivary glands. Am J Surg. 1970;120:432-8.
53. Spiro RH, Huvos AG, Berk R, Strong EW. Mucoepidermoid carcinoma of salivary gland origin: A clinicopathologic study of 367 cases. Am J Surg. 1978;136:461-8.
54. O'Brien CJ, Soong SJ, Herrera GA, Urist MM, Maddox WA. Malignant salivary tumors–analysis of prognostic factors and survival. Head Neck Surg. 1986;9:82-92.
55. Maciejewski A, Szymczyk C, Wierzgon J. Outcome of surgery for adenoid cystic carcinoma of head and neck region. J Cranio-Maxillofac Surg. 2002;30:59-61.
56. Tomich CE. Adenoid Cystic Carcinoma. Ellis GL, Auclair PL, Gnepp DR (Eds). Surgical Pathology of the Salivary glands. WB Saunders, Philadelphia. 1991; 19:333-49.
57. Kim KH, Sung MW. Adenoid cystic carcinoma of the head and neck. Arch Otolaryngol Head Neck Surg. 1994;120:721-6.
58. Spiro RH, Huvos AG, Strong EW. Cancer of the parotid gland: A clinicopathologic study of 288 primary cases. Am J Surg. 1975;130:452-9.
59. Eneroth CM. Salivary gland tumors in the parotid gland, submandibular gland and the palate region, Cancer. 1971;27:1415-8.
60. Batsakis JG. Tumors of the head and neck–Clinical and pathological considerations; 2nd edn. Williams and Wilkins, Baltimore. 1979;1.
61. Hanna EY, Suen JY. Malignant tumors of the salivary glands. Myers EN, Suen JY, Myers JN, Hanna EY, (Eds). Cancer of the head and neck, 4th edn. Saunders. 21:475-510.
62. Bell RB, Dierks EJ, Homer L, Potter BE. Management and outcome of patients with malignant salivary gland tumors. J Oral Maxillofac Surg. 2005;63:917-28.
63. Spiro RH, Armstrong J, Harrison L, Geller NL, Lin SY, Strong EW. Carcinoma of major salivary glands: Major trends. Arch Otolaryngol Head Neck Surg. 1989;115:316-21.
64. Matsuba HM, Spector GJ, Thawley Se, Simpson JR, Mauney M, Pikul FJ. Adenoid cystic salivary gland carcinoma: A Histopathologic review of treatment failure patterns, Cancer. 1986;57:519-24.
65. Adam Maciejewski, Cezary Szymczyk, Janusz Wierzgon. Outcome of surgery for adenoid cystic carcinoma of head and neck region. J Cranio-Maxillofacial Surg. 2002;30:59-61.

66. Witten J, Hybert F, Hansen HS. Treatment of malignant tumors in the parotid glands, Cancer. 1990;65:2515-20.
67. Auclair PL, Ellis GL. Acinic cell adenocarcinoma. Ellis GL, Auclair PL, Gnepp DR (Eds). Surgical Pathology of the Salivary glands. WB Saunders, Philadelphia. 1991;17:318-32.
68. Yih WY, Kratochvil FJ, Stewart J. Intraoral minor salivary gland neoplasms: Review of 213 cases. J Oral Maxillofac Surg. 2005;63:805-10.
69. Spiro RH, Huvos AG, Strong EW. Cancer of the parotid gland: A clinicopathologic study of 288 primary cases. Am J Surg. 1975;130:452-9.
70. Spiro RH, Huvos AG, Strong EW. Acinic cell carcinoma of salivary origin: A clinicopathologic study of cases. Cancer. 1978;41:924-35.
71. Hickman RE, Cawson RA, Duffy SW. The prognosis of specific types of salivary gland tumors. Cancer. 1984;54:1620-24.
72. Levitt SH, McHugh RB, Gomez-Marin O, Hyams VJ, Soules EH, Strong EW, et al. Clinical staging system for cancer of the salivary gland: a retrospective study. Cancer 1981;47:2712-24.
73. Douglas Gnepp, Bruce Wenig. Malignant Mixed Tumors. Ellis GL, Auclair PL, Gnepp DR, editors. Surgical Pathology of the Salivary Glands. WB Saunders, Philadelphia. 1991;20:350-68.
74. Spiro RH, Huvos AG, Strong EW. Malignant mixed tumor of salivary origin: A clinicopathologic study of 146 cases, Cancer. 1977;39:388-96.
75. Tortoledo ME, Luna MA, Batsakis JG. Carcinomas ex pleomorphic adenoma and malignant mixed tumors. Arch Otolaryngol. 1984;110:172-6.
76. Nagao K, Matsuzaki O, saiga H, Sugano I, Shigematsu H, Kaneko T, Katoh T, Kitamura T. Histopathologic studies on carcinoma in pleomorphic adenoma of the parotid gland, Cancer. 1981;48:113-21.
77. LiVolsi VA, Perzin KH. Malignant mixed tumors arising in salivary glands. Carcinomas arising in benign mixed tumors. A clinicopathologic study, Cancer. 1977;39:2209-30.
78. Hickman RE, Cawson RA, Duffy SW. The prognosis of specific types of salivary gland tumors. Cancer. 1984;54:1620-24.
79. Stephen J, Batsakis JG, Luna MA, von der Heyden U, Byers RM. True malignant mixed tumors (Carcinosarcoma) of salivary glands. Oral Surg Oral Med Oral Pathol 1986;61:597-602.
80. Thomas KM, Hutt MSR, Borgstein J. Salivary gland tumors in Malawi. Cancer. 1980;46:2328-34.
81. Auclair PL, Ellis GL. Primary squamous cell carcinoma. Ellis GL, Auclair PL, Gnepp DR, (Eds). Surgical Pathology of the Salivary Glands. WB Saunders, Philadelphia. 1991;21:369-78.
82. Shemen LJ, Huvos AG, Spiro RH. Squamous cell carcinoma of salivary gland origin. Head Neck Surg. 1987;9:235-40.
83. Reddy SP, Marks JE. Treatment of locally advanced, high-grade, malignant tumors of major salivary glands. Laryngoscope. 1988;98:450-4.

84. Auclair PL, Ellis GL. Clear cell carcinoma. Ellis GL, Auclair PL, Gnepp DR, editors. Surgical Pathology of the Salivary Glands. WB Saunders, Philadelphia. 1991;22:379-89.
85. Corio RL. Epithelial - Myoepithelial carcinoma. Ellis GL, Auclair PL, Gnepp DR (eds). Surgical Pathology of the Salivary Glands. WB Saunders, Philadelphia. 1991;24:412-21.
86. Corio RL, Sciubba JJ, Brannon RB, Batsakis JG. Epithelial-myoepithelial carcinoma of intercalated duct origin. Oral Surg Oral Med Oral Pathol. 1982;53:280-7.
87. Batsakis JG. Tumors of the head and neck – Clinical and pathological considerations 2nd edn. Williams and Wilkins, Baltimore. 1979;1.
88. Luna MA, Ordonez NG, Mackay B, Batsakis JG, Guillamondegui O. Salivary epithelial-myoepithelial carcinoma of intercalated ducts: A clinical, electron microscopic, and immunocytochemical study. Oral Surg Oral Med Oral Pathol 1985;59:482-90.
89. Stiernberg CM, Batsakis JG, Bailey BJ, Clark WD. Epithelial-myoepithelial carcinoma of the parotid gland. Otolaryngol Head Neck Surg. 1986;94:240-2.
90. Ferreria JL, Maurino N, Michael E, Ratinoff M, Rubio E. Surgery of the parotid region: A new approach. J Oral and Maxillofac Surg. 1990;48:803-7.
91. Farrior JB, Santini H. facial nerve identification in children. Otolaryngol Head Neck Surg. 1985;93:173.
92. Hanna EY, Lee S, Fan CY, Suen JY. Benign neoplasms of the salivary glands. Haughley BH, (Edn) Cummings Otolaryngology Head and Neck Surgery, 4th edn. Elsevier Mosby publication, 2005.pp.1348-77.
93. Meningaud JP, Bertolus C, Bertrand JC. Parotidectomy: Assessment of A surgical technique including facelift incision and SMAS advancement. Journal of Cranio-Maxillofacial Surg. 2006;34:34-7.
94. Shah JP. Color atlas of operative techniques in Head and Neck Surgery. Wolfe Medical Publications, England. pp.117-33.
95. Johns M, Nachlas N. Salivary gland tumors Paperella, Shumrick, Gluckman, Meyerhoff (Eds) Otolaryngology. WB Saunders Company, Philafelphia. 1991; 20(3):2099–127.

Surgical management of parotid neoplasms

chapter 12

The management of salivary gland neoplasms, both benign and malignant, is primarily surgical. Management of salivary gland malignancy, especially in advanced-stage disease, close or positive margins or ominous histology, may be achieved by combined modality therapy including surgery and postoperative radiotherapy. Surgical treatment of the primary site for both major and minor glands has not changed much in past few decades. The facial nerve should be spared as far as possible and if sacrificed it should be reconstructed immediately with interpositional nerve graft in almost all the patients.[1] Small (T_1–T_2) tumors of the superficial lobe of the parotid gland that are located lateral to the plane of the facial nerve may be adequately treated with a superficial parotidectomy. Larger tumors and tumors involving the deep lobe of the parotid gland usually require a total parotidectomy. In case facial nerve is sacrificed in management of malignant tumors, surgical margins on both the distal and the proximal nerve stumps should be checked because of the possibility of perineural spread for some distance from the area of the primary tumor. Tumors extending beyond the confines of the parotid gland may require resection of surrounding structures, including the skin, mandibular ramus, and masseter muscle; infratemporal fossa dissection; and/or subtotal petrosectomy.[2]

Patient preparation

The hair is clipped and shaved in front of the ear up to one finger breadth above the pinna and also behind the ear if hairline encroaches upon the mastoid process. Patient receives an antiseptic soap facial scrub and a shampoo bath night before the surgery. Parts are prepared with surgical scrub. Induction of general anesthesia can be achieved by using short acting muscle relaxants but a longer acting muscle relaxant is avoided and hypotensive anesthesia is requested unless contraindicated by the patient's general health. It is preferred that the side of the face to be operated is not covered by drapes to visualize the twitching of the facial muscles. The external auditory meatus is plugged with vaseline gauze to prevent blood from filling the canal.

Skin incision and exposure of the gland[3]

This part of the procedure is common to all the resection procedures unless skin is being excised because it is involved by the tumor. The ideal incision should combine good exposure with the best ultimate cosmetic result.

Gutierrez had laid down guidelines for gaining access to the parotid gland in 1903. The incision had a temporal extension, a preauricular component and a limb extending on to the neck in one of the skin creases **(Figure 12.1)**. Subsequently, Adson and Ott, Martin, Wolf attempted to improvise this incision. Adson does not consider using the temporal incision line for exposure of the parotid gland. All the incisions had a common feature, the vertical component that extends from the retroauricular region into the neck, allowing dissection of the lower anterior portion of the neck. However, the chief drawback of these incisions was esthetics in case of development of a keloid.

Yoel and Bilesio had suggested a modification to Gutierrez's incision that has been used previously with good results. However, the drawback was that, in case of delayed healing esthetics would be hampered.

Similarly, Redon and Vaillant and Laudenbach have proposed an incision line similar to that proposed by Adson **(Figure 12.2)**.

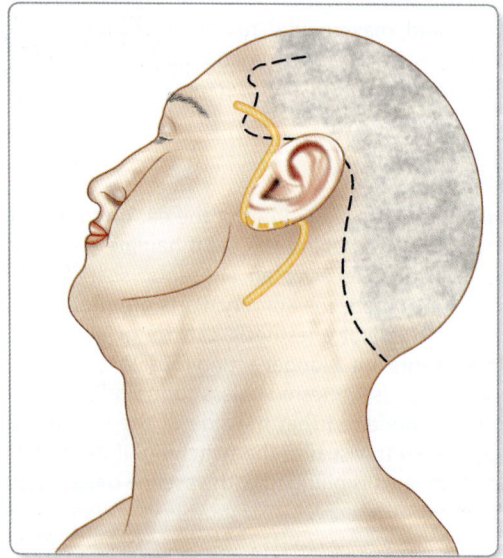

Figure 12.1 Gutierrez incision

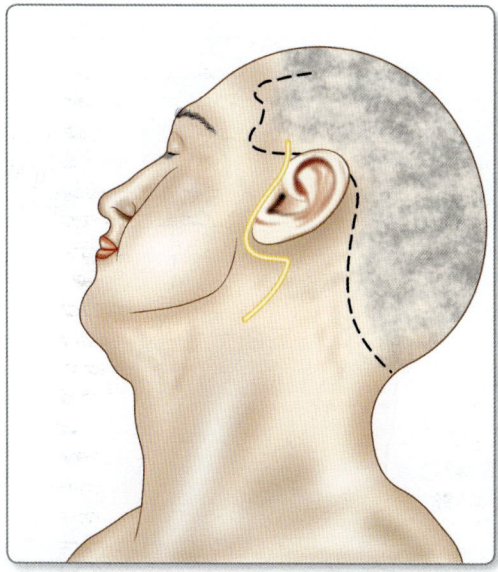

Figure 12.2 Redon and Vaillant and Laudenbach incision

In addition to the above modification, Adson and Ott have described a 'Y' shaped incision with a preauricular sector, a postauricular sector and a cervical incision line, that splits off from the site of union of the first two branches **(Figure 12.3)**.

The advantage of this incision is improved esthetics because it lacks a temporal incision line. However, the drawback of this incision is that it impairs dissection. Also one section of the incision is located in the carotid region.

Samengo, 1961, proposed a similar incision having a preauricular, a postauricular and a neck extension in the incision line **(Figure 12.4)**.

Finally, in 1967 Appiani described a technique that involves an incision within the lower portion of the scalp and is hidden by the hair instead of the vertical incision line. The benefit of this incision is better esthetics because the incision is masked by hair. However, the temporal extension of this incision is short and this impairs access to the anterior portion of the gland **(Figure 12.5)**.

Ferreria JL et al have further suggested modification to Appiani's incision. They have extended the temporal incision line but not beyond the hairline. The major advantage of this incision is that it provides a better access to the anterior portion of the parotid gland without compromising esthetics.

178 Salivary gland pathologies

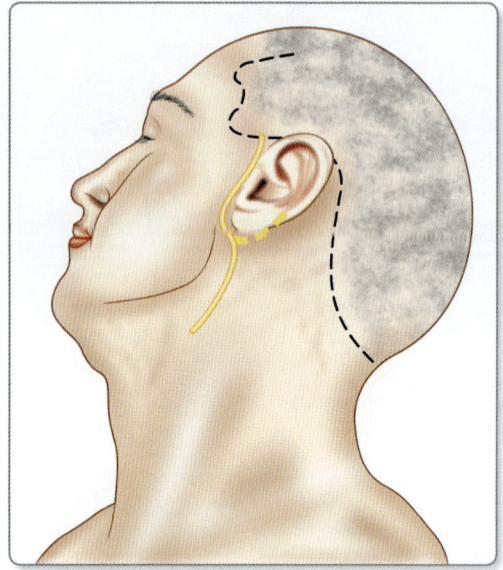

Figure 12.3 Adson and Ott incision

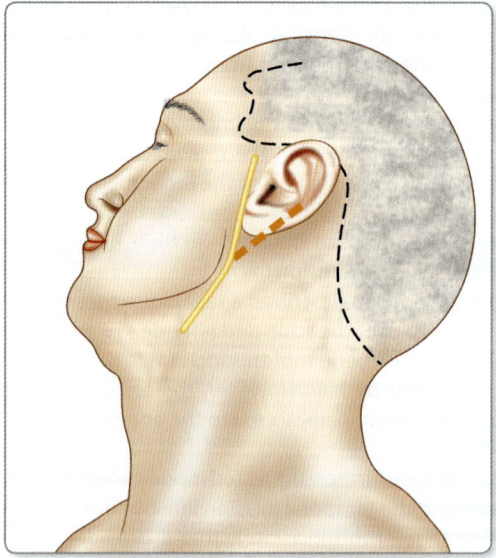

Figure 12.4 Samengo incision

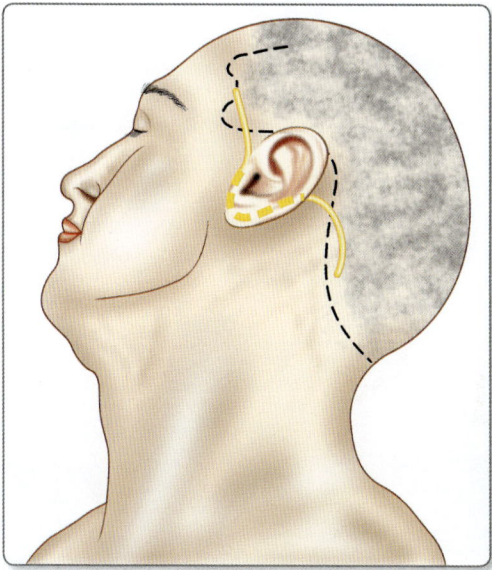

Figure 12.5 Appiani's incision

Dissection may be compromised only in cases of very large tumors of the gland. One more improvization in the incision line is rounding off of the angles where the incision line changes direction. This modification reduces the incidence of dehiscence and salivary fistula formation. In case a radical neck dissection is to be carried out in conjunction with the parotidectomy, the same incision can be increased without compromising the vascularity of the flaps.

Farrior et al recommended a single curved incision 1.5 to 2.0 cm below the mandible and extending over the mastoid region 1.5 cm behind the postauricular crease. The preauricular crease used in adults is avoided because of the superficial location of the facial nerve and possibility of facial nerve damage during flap elevation.[4]

The standard incision is a modified Blair's incision **(Figure 12.6)** wherein the skin incision is placed in a preauricular crease and extends superiorly to the level of the root of the helix. The incision extends inferiorly around the lobule of ear over the mastoid tip. It gently curves down along the sternocleidomastoid muscle and then slightly forward in a natural crease in the upper neck.[5]

Benign tumors of the parotid gland are classically removed via an incision extending to the neck without reconstruction of the parotid bed.

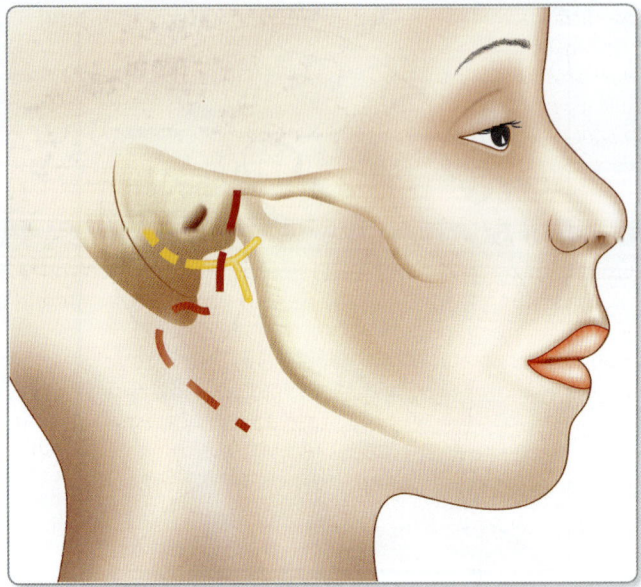

Figure 12.6 Modified Blair's incision in adult
(*Modified from Rankow:* Diseases of salivary glands)

Two consequences are usual: a conspicuous scar and a deep hollow dorsal to the mandible. These drawbacks can be prevented or reduced by using a facelift approach (Appiani and Delfino, 1984; Ferreria et al, 1990) with a superficial musculoaponeurotic system (SMAS) advancement flap (Bonanno and Casson, 1992). Despite its proven safety and its relevance regarding the cosmetic outcome, the SMAS-lifting technique is not a routine procedure for many surgeons.[6]

Identification of the facial nerve

This has been previously described in the section on applied anatomy of the parotid gland.

Tumor resection

Every reasonable attempt must be made to achieve negative resection margins at the time of ablative surgery.[1] Depending on the pathological extent of the tumor it can take several forms:[7]
a. Local excision of the parotid gland

b. Superficial parotidectomy with preservation of the facial nerve
c. Functional superficial parotidectomy
d. Total parotidectomy with preservation of the facial nerve
e. Radical parotidectomy with or without neck dissection in continuity
f. Parotidomandibulectomy
g. Temporoparotidectomy.

Local excision of parotid gland[8]

This surgical procedure is carried out for excision of Warthin's tumor. It can be carried out when the tumor is present on the tail of the parotid gland and the maximum dimension of the tumor is less than 3.5 cm. Hence, there is enough normal gland tissue separating the tumor from the main duct and the anterior-upper portion of the parotid gland to allow excision. After resection of the tumor with adequate surrounding normal tissue most of the parotid gland can be preserved. Most parotid lymph nodes are in the

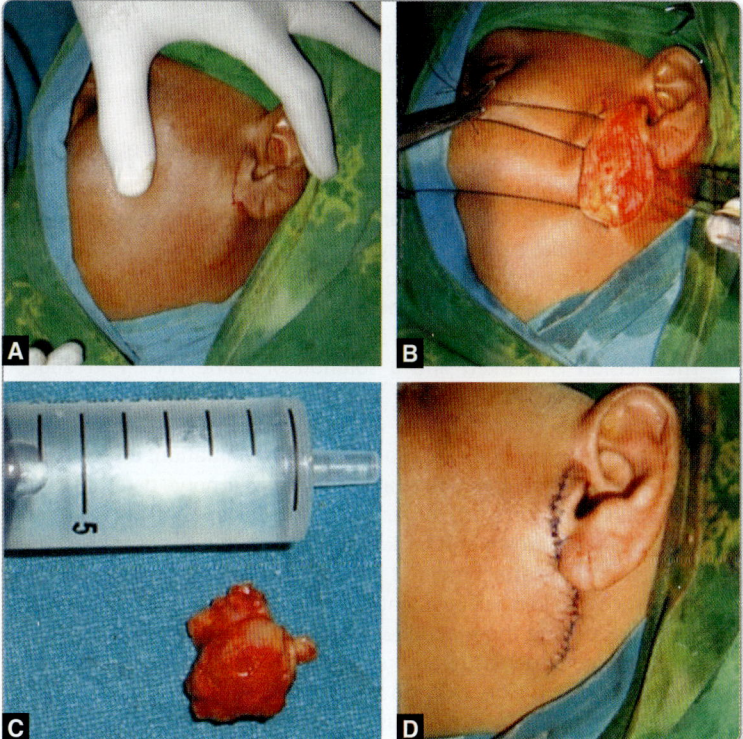

Figures 12.7A to D (A) Parotid exposure through Blair's incision; (B) Identification of tumor mass; (C) Excised specimen; (D) Closure

postero-inferior portion of the gland with some in the pre-auricular region. Warthin's tumor rarely occurs in the preauricular region and hence adequate resection of the gland along with the associated lymph nodes is possible by local excision of the parotid tail.

An 'S' shaped incision is marked with the upper end of the 'S' slightly short of the ear lobe. The flap is raised to show the anterior and inferior borders of the gland. The marginal mandibular branch of the facial nerve is located on the anterior border of the masseter muscle where it exits from the gland. The nerve is dissected in a retrograde direction until the cervicofacial bifurcation of the facial nerve is exposed. The retromandibular vein can also be used to locate the marginal mandibular nerve as it lies deep to the facial nerve and enters the deep lobe of the parotid gland. The anterior-upper portion of the parotid gland is preserved along with the stenson's duct. The tumor is excised along with a margin of normal glandular structure and the overlying parotid lymph nodes. Several lymph nodes are located in the tail of the parotid gland and at the junction of the posterior border of the gland and anterior border of the sternomastoid muscle. In some of them either microadenomas or tumors occupying the whole node may be found on microscopic examination. Hence, the tumor along with the lymph nodes should be resected to prevent recurrence.

Parotidectomy with preservation of the facial nerve

It is also known as superficial parotidectomy or conservative parotidectomy. However both the terminologies are inappropriate to the tumor surgery. The term superficial parotidectomy is inaccurate because it implies the existence of a superficial and deep lobe connected by an isthmus which is no more accepted. However superficial parotidectomy may be used to imply surgical excision of the gland superficial to the facial nerve.

The incision is marked and a solution of saline with 1 in 200000 parts adrenaline is injected under the skin over the parotid, anterior to the external ear and close to the external auditory canal. A solution of adrenaline with lignocaine can also be used for infiltration, but care must be taken to avoid deep injection to avoid risk of facial nerve paralysis during the procedure.[9] Incision starts within the hair line above and anterior to the auricle and is taken down and back to the free margin of the tragus. Then, it passes around the attachment of the ear lobe in a gentle curve over the mastoid process to join a convenient skin crease passing down and forward into the neck behind the mandible. Part or whole of the crease line may be used depending on the exposure required. Persistent edema will occur postoperatively if it is extended too far posteriorly beneath the ear lobe.

The incision in the neck crease is deepened first exposing and dividing the platysma which extends into the anterior end of the wound until the deep fascia is reached. The deep fascia is seen as a white sheet and is easily identifiable as it is thick and dense at the angle of the mandible.

The greater auricular nerve which lies along a line joining the midpoint of the posterior border of the sternomastoid to the angle of the mandible should be identified and preserved at this stage. This nerve crosses the surface of the muscle to lie in the wound approximately 1 cm below and 1 cm in front of the lobe of the ear immediately below the deep fascia and just posterior to the external jugular vein. Sometimes it may even appear in the subcutaneous tissue as the incision is placed and should be carefully preserved in the flap. It will be seen to branch over the surface of the gland and two or more branches should be followed and then divided. The nerve with the branches attached is tucked under the lower edge of the wound to keep it moist. One or two sutures can be used in retaining the nerve in its proper position.

Once the deep fascia has been identified rest of the wound is deepened to this level and skin reflected forward from it. There will be relatively little bleeding and the branches of the facial nerve will not be endangered as they lie deep to the deep fascia at the anterior border of the gland. As the zygomatic bone is approached some subcutaneous fat should be left on the fascia because here the branches lie more superficially as they emerge from the upper part of the parotid. They do not penetrate deep fascia till they reach the anterior border of the masseter. The branches will be visible through the translucent fascia as they emerge from the anterior border of the gland. They may be uncovered by opening the fascia with thin-bladed, blunt-pointed scissors and gently separating its layers. Even if the trunk of the nerve is to be identified and traced forward into the gland it is helpful to identify some of the branches as they emerge from it anteriorly, because the expanding neoplasm will have pushed them aside and their paths may take unexpected twists and turns, making it advantageous to work from both ends of the nerve. As each branch is identified it is labeled by under-running it with a length of black silk, the ends of which are clamped in mosquito artery forceps.

The main trunk of the nerve lies at a surprising depth from the surface in the angle between the bony external auditory canal and the anterior surface of the mastoid process. It is found by first separating the lower pole of the gland from the anterior border of the sternomastoid and then from the mastoid process and the cartilaginous part of the external auditory meatus. The loose connective tissue close to the cartilage is relatively avascular, but the tiny occipital branch of the posterior auricular artery which runs across the front of the mastoid process is often a nuisance, as the cartilaginous part is uncovered. Systematic, careful hemostasis is maintained or visibility will be impaired. The wound is deepened anterior to the margin of the sternomastoid and the lower pole is dissected free as far forward as the

184 Salivary gland pathologies

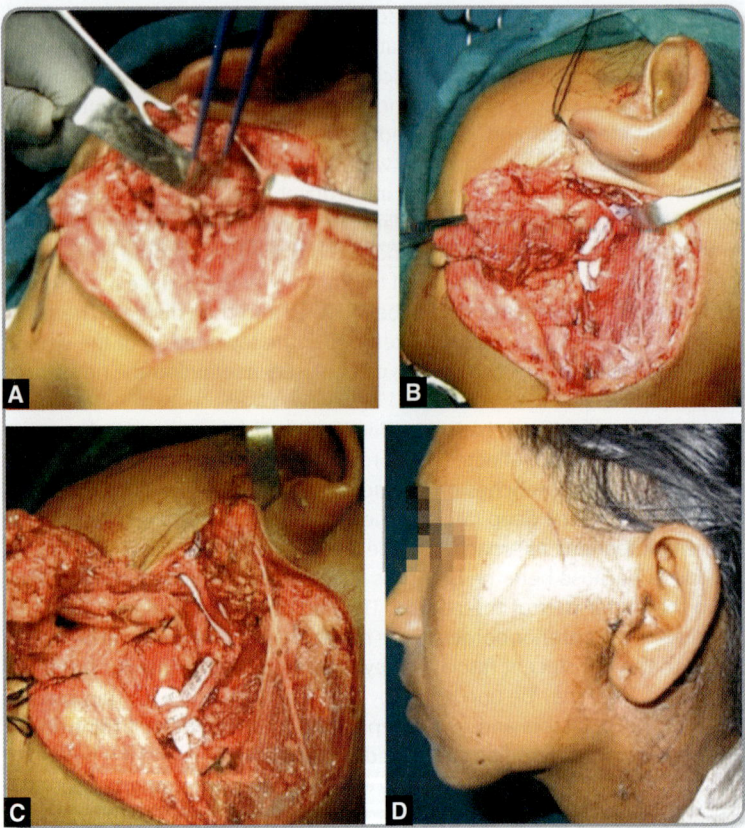

Figures 12.8A to D (A) Parotid exposure through Blair's incision; (B) Identification of facial nerve; (C) Superficial parotidectomy; (D) Postoperative scar

external jugular, uncovering the posterior belly of the digastric muscle. The vein should not be divided and tied at this stage because this will increase the venous engorgement of the parotid and the ooze from its divided tissues.

Neither should the lower pole be raised further forward because the branches of the facial nerve often pass superficial to the vein and emerge from the gland anterior to it. Indeed the cervical branch tends to lie near the posterior facial vein in this part. The parotid is retracted forward as the dissection proceeds and the pointed, lower extremity of the tragal cartilage will be uncovered. Due to the presence of this pointed terminal portion, the auricular cartilage is also termed as "pointer cartilage". Approximately

1 cm deep to the cartilage and lying inferior and anterior is the main trunk of the facial nerve. Immediately deep to the cartilage is the edge of the bony-part of the external auditory canal. The nerve emerges in the angle between the tympanic bone and the anterior border of the mastoid process and just superior to the upper border of the posterior belly of the digastric. The interval between the tympanic bone and the muscle is a short one, but the nerve may lie either high or low within it. Further, it is covered by the tympanomastoid fascia which stretches between the back of the gland and the tympanomastoid fissure, and being quite tough, often needs to be cut with scissors. Where possible the edge of the fascia should be raised and the underlying tissue separated by blunt dissection until the nerve is seen as a white cords some 2 to 3 mm thick. The stylomastoid branch of the posterior auricular artery passes superficial to the nerve to enter the stylomastoid foramen. Rough instrumentation can tear this small vessel causing hemorrhage at this critical stage. Damage to this vessel should also be avoided as it supplies a nutrient branch to the nerve. Though the nerve is deeply placed it is not more so than the plane of the posterior belly of the digastric. Dissection deep to this level carries the operator onto the internal jugular vein and if pursued above and anterior to the site of the nerve may uncover the styloid process. The facial nerve and its branches are invested by loose connective tissue and lie in tunnels within the parotid into which the tips of the blades of curved mosquito artery forceps may be insinuated. The blades are then opened a little to stretch the tissues and raised, so as to lift the gland substance off the surface of the nerve, a short length of which may then be exposed by cutting through the gland with scissors. Alternatively a scalpel is used, introducing a small no. 11 or no. 15 blade into the tunnel with the back of the blade facing the nerve so as to cut away from it. At all times when a cut is made the adjacent nerve must be seen clearly.

Almost immediately the nerve trunk starts to travel laterally within the parotid to pass around the posterior border of the mandible and just below the neck of the condyle. As it does so it splits into an upper temporofacial and a lower cervicofacial division. Because its path is ascending towards the surgeon its exposure and the dissection of the gland is awkward. Nevertheless the procedure must not be hastened nor executed too boldly lest one or more of the branches are cut at a point where they lie more superficially. Soon they turn forward parallel to the surface of the gland and progress is less difficult. Generally it is better to follow the lower division first and trace the cervical or the marginal mandibular branch anteriorly to a point in front of the parotid. In this way the lower pole can be mobilized completely. Then by progressing upwards, branch by branch further mobilization can be achieved.

Tissue adjacent to tumor is compressed into a thin capsule. Where the tumor reaches the surface of the gland some overlying subcutaneous fat should be left to cover it as the flap is raised. Penetration on the deep surface will bring it into contact with the muscle such as Masseter or loose connective tissue. The former can be excised in continuity with the mass; the latter should be divided under direct vision some little distance from the tumor and allowed to collapse on to its surface.

In general branches of the nerve which pass over the surface of the tumor but still lie within a sheath of loose connective tissue may be safely separated and their continuity preserved, providing care is exercised not to break the surface of the tumor and seed the wound. Those which pass into the tumor must be divided and the point at which they emerge identified and divided again. Both ends are 'tagged' for subsequent repair. At least one branch above the part of the gland to be excised should be traced out to avoid damaging it unnecessarily.

Filamentous structures passing horizontally or radiating from the region of the main trunk are likely to be nerves and should be conserved. The branches decrease in diameter as they are traced peripherally in contrast to the main duct which increases in size to reach 2 to 3 mm in cross-section as it emerges from the gland anteriorly. Further it passes diagonally upwards and forwards. Blood vessels, except for the transverse facial generally run up from below, and, unlike nerves, have elasticity, so that with care they can be distinguished. Branches from the great auricular nerve differ from those of the facial by remaining on the surface of the gland as they are traced posteriorly.

Interconnecting branches joining two peripheral branches vertically may be encountered and if possible should be conserved. In general the nerves pass superficial to the retromandibular vein but some may pass deep to it. Careful mobilization of both nerve and vein with division and ligation of the latter is necessary. Tiny vessels should be sealed with diathermy by accurately grasping them with fine artery forceps and touching briefly with the electrode, avoiding damage to adjacent nerves.

Complications

1. Facial paresis or paralysis often result from poor technique and failure to preserve small nerve branches.
2. Bleeding and hematoma formation, which can significantly compromise the airway.
3. Rarely, persistent salivary leakage or sialocele formation occurs.
4. Frey's syndrome.
5. Skin flap necrosis.

Functional superficial parotidectomy[10]

It involves the preservation of gland function by preservation of the Stenson's duct. The preservation of gland function depends on the extent of tissue removed. In superficial parotidectomy, whether excretory function of the deep lobe of parotid gland can be preserved will depend on the relationship of the duct with the facial nerve. If the duct is superficial to the buccal branch, its preservation is contraindicated because it will cause a hindrance in efficient surgical procedure. However, as much as 91.4% of ducts are deep to the facial nerve. Hence it can be performed routinely.

In this, after raising the skin and subcutaneous tissue flap exposure of the parotid gland is achieved up to the anterior border of the parotid gland. The parotid duct (Stenson's duct) is identified passing on the Masseter muscle. It is located on an imaginary line joining the base of the ear lobe to the vermilion border of the upper lip. This is used for the identification of the buccal branch of the facial nerve. Once the Stenson's duct is located, dissection and ligation of the duct is avoided unless it is located superficial to the buccal branches of the facial nerve.

After this step, facial nerve identification and preservation is carried out following which superficial lobe containing the tumor is removed. After removal of the superficial lobe, the facial nerve remains over the surface of the deep lobe with the main parotid duct in continuity, unless previously cut.

Advantages of functional superficial parotidectomy
1. It is a simpler surgery than conservative superficial parotidectomy.
2. It preserves partial function of the parotid gland.
3. It avoids the influence of subsequent gland atrophy on facial contour.
4. It decreases postoperative complications.

Partial superficial parotidectomy

In recent years, partial superficial parotidectomy has emerged as a more conservative approach than superficial parotidectomy in the management of parotid tumors. In this procedure only the tumor-bearing area of the gland parenchyma is removed. The main trunk of the facial nerve is identified and the facial nerve branches that are adjacent to the tumor site are dissected and preserved with no need for any more extensive facial nerve dissection. Thus, few branches of the facial nerve are dissected and less normal parotid tissue is removed.

The advantage of this procedure over superficial parotidectomy is relatively low incidence of Frey's syndrome. The reported incidence of this complication is 4.8%.[11] In addition, better gland function is preserved due to more parenchyma that is left back.[12]

Intraoral deep lobe tumor excision[13]

It is used in removal of select few benign tumors by using transoral approach. It is indicated in deep lobe benign tumors smaller than 5 cm.

Under general anesthesia, a mouth gag is inserted to expose the palate and tonsillar region. The tumor should be easily visible, displacing the superior portion of the tonsil and soft palate medially. An incision is made over the most prominent aspect of the swelling in the tonsil and palate area, extending above and below the apparent location of the tumor. The initial incision can be made with cautery or knife. Meticulous hemostasis should be maintained at every stage of the procedure.

After the initial incision is given, the constrictor muscle is identified. The dissection is continued through thinned constrictor muscle. A clamp is placed in a plane deep to the constrictor muscle and superficial to the tumor and the muscle is divided above and below the tumor.

The tumor capsule is then visible. No retractors are placed on the capsule and pressure on the neck often assists in removal of the tumor. With blunt instrumentation, any fascial connections from the tumor in to the adjacent bed are removed and the tumor is delivered into the mouth. Any vascular connections to the tumor should be cauterized and meticulous hemostasis should be achieved. The superior and inferior portions of the wound are closed with interrupted sutures. The middle portion of the wound is left open to heal secondarily.

Complications

1. Tumor rupture
2. Incomplete removal
3. Uncontrolled hemorrhage

Total parotidectomy with or without facial nerve preservation

An anatomically complete ablation of every scrap of the parotid will confer no particular benefit on the patient, nor indeed is it practical. A more complete removal than superficial parotidectomy with preservation of facial nerve will be practiced where a slow growing mass, not clinically malignant, is present in the deep part. The facial nerve is dissected out first, actually dividing only those superficial tissues necessary to display the nerve. It is then mobilized completely from the gland and the deep portion of the gland with its contained tumor is removed. The other indication for total parotidectomy is where a small neoplasm is recognized on clinical grounds as malignant and to secure the necessary margin to contain the lesion, it is decided to remove the gland without attempting to dissect out the nerve. Careful consideration must be given to the advisability of biopsy and frozen section before the main trunk of the nerve is divided.

A large, slowly growing tumor of the deep part of the parotid may present as a swelling of the soft palate. Characteristically this becomes more obvious when the patient says 'ah' and raises the soft palate. On examination under an anesthetic it is apparent that it is a large mass which has enlarged from its lateral aspect. A neoplasm of a palatal mucous gland protrudes far more into the oral cavity and its periphery is easier to define by palpation. Indeed, if entirely within the soft palate it will be relatively mobile under the examining fingers.

A neoplasm of the deep part of the parotid enters the soft palate through the interval between the styloid process and the back of the mandible. It is often of dumbbell shape with the isthmus lying in this gap. The lateral portion is usually sufficiently large to indent the gland appreciably on a sialogram, as is well shown in a CAT scan.

Where the involvement of the soft palate is considerable the biopsy may be performed on this aspect. It is best done under general anesthesia with a local infiltration of vasoconstrictor so that the nature of the incised tissues is not obscured by hemorrhage. It is likely that the lesions will be separated from the mucous membrane by a layer of palatal muscle. This must be

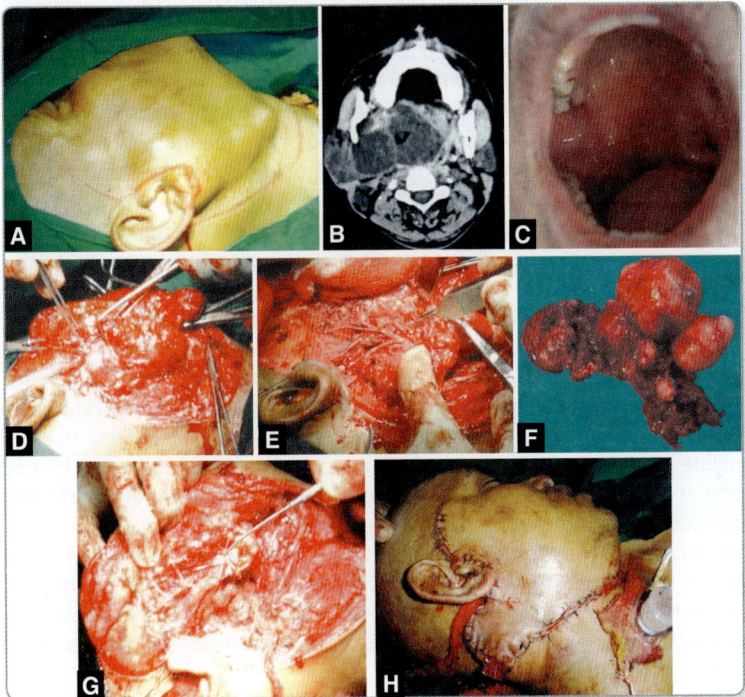

Figures 12.9A to H (A) Blair incision marked; (B) CT scan showing dumbbell tumor; (C) Involvement of deep lobe: shift of soft palate and uvula to the left; (D) Exposure; (E) Facial nerve dissection; (F) Specimen showing involvement of submandibular gland as well; (G) Postoperative defect; (H) Closure

divided before taking the specimen or the fragment will not contain tumor tissue. Having confirmed its benign nature the definitive operation may take place when the wound scar should be excised in continuity with the main mass.

A skin flap is raised in the usual way but the incision in a neck skin crease is continued as far forward as the first molar region. The facial nerve is dissected out leaving a layer of glandular tissue over the surface of the tumor. The periosteum is then divided at the lower border of the angle of the mandible and the masseter elevated from the bone. A vertical cut similar to that used for a vertical subsigmoid osteotomy is made in the mandible from the sigmoid notch to the lower border skirting just behind the mandibular foramen. The medial pterygoid is freed from the posterior fragment so that it can be displaced forwards lateral to the anterior fragment. This opens up the interval between the mandible and the styloid process through which the tumor has passed. As an alternative the mandible may be sectioned in the premolar region anterior to the mental foramen and the angle retracted upwards.

The lower pole of the parotid is mobilized and the surface of the digastric and stylohyoid muscles followed back to their origins. The stylohyoid muscle may be divided close to the styloid process and turned forward. The external carotid artery will be encountered emerging above the muscles and should be divided. The origin of the facial artery should be identified to check the identity of the vessel.

The facial nerve branches are gathered into two bundles relating to the upper and lower divisions and each is supported on tapes. As the parotid gland and the tumor are freed the lower bundle may be slipped under the lower pole so that the mass is raised up between the two bundles. Alternatively the gland may be brought out below both bundles, whichever maneuver is more convenient. At this stage the mouth which has been prepared at the beginning with antiseptic solution is uncovered and entered. A solution of adrenaline 1: 200 000 in saline is injected into the soft palate over the swelling and a vertical incision, circumscribing any biopsy scar, is made. Its edges are undermined, leaving a thin layer of muscle and connective tissue over the tumor. By working through both wounds the mass can be freed mostly under direct vision. Great care must be exercised above and particularly behind the lesion for fear of damaging the internal jugular vein or internal carotid artery, both of which lie deep to the styloid process. Blind cutting is therefore not permissible and the tissues must always be divided under direct vision.

Following removal of the mass the wound is irrigated and the oral tissues closed with care using 4/0 chromic catgut as a continuous suture. The drapes are replaced over the mouth, gloves changed and the mandibular fragments wired together. The preauricular wound is closed in layers with drainage in the usual way.

Parotidectomy using SMAS plane for dissection[6]

The SMAS flap is undoubtedly the user-friendliest flap to fill the soft-tissue defect in the dorsal part of the cheek. The dissection is easy and rapid, provided it is done in the parotid region. It is even easier after a hydrodissection and using spatulated scissors. Undermining has to be carried out at the level of the parotid aponeurosis. The grayish color of the parotid gland contrasts with the yellow one of the SMAS. The trick is to use the SMAS flap as a membrane for guided tissue regeneration. The tip of the SMAS flap alone is too small to fill the entire defect. Actually, it is essential that the hematoma below the SMAS becomes organized by scar tissue thus filling the parotid bed. Sometimes the tumor is too close to the SMAS layer and a hole has to be made in order to remove the tumor with a free margin of tissue around. This holds true also for pleomorphic adenomas as pseudocapsule-free regions, satellite nodules, and pseudopodia are frequent (Stennert et al., 2004). Simple enucleation enhances the risk of recurrence (45% in some series; Paris et al, 2004). Nevertheless, we have to recognize with Donovan and Conley (1984) that close dissection (at least in part) is often the reality at the time of the operation, e.g. in very anterior tumors. When a hole through the SMAS layer has to be made, repairing it with a few sutures is sufficient. But the SMAS flap also has positive functional consequences.

The advantages of this flap are that exposure of the gland is sufficient and the dissection is easy to perform. There is no donor-site morbidity, minimum additional operating time, and no extra cost. It seems to decrease the incidence of Frey's syndrome. The speed of the recovery of the facial nerve has been highlighted in the literature. And the main result of this article is that it is more satisfactory from the patient's point of view.

Parotidomandibulectomy[7]

Parotidomandibulectomy is indicated where there is invasion of the mandible by a malignant neoplasm and where it is hoped that in relation to its other surfaces an adequate margin can be obtained. The face and mouth are prepared and a skin flap raised, as for excision of a benign neoplasm of the deep part of the parotid. The gland is mobilized posteriorly and inferiorly and the main trunk of the facial nerve identified. As many branches are dissected out as is possible without encroaching upon the necessary margin about the neoplasm. Section of the main trunk and sacrifice of the whole nerve may well be necessary. The tissues are divided anterior to the line of excision and all the peripheral branches labeled particularly those to be cut. The capsule of the temporomandibular joint is opened and the condyle mobilized. The masseter is separated from the zygomatic arch and the mandible divided in the third molar region. The parotid and mandibular ramus are tilted up and forward and separated from the styloid process and its attached muscles. Any branches of the cervicofacial division which have been conserved are gathered into a bundle with a loop of tape and slipped down over the specimen. Further elevation of the ramus is then possible and a finger can be passed up medial to the medial pterygoid muscle defining its origin from the tuberosity and the pterygoid plate. The blades of a pair of stout scissors are passed along the finger to cut first the fibers attached to the tuberosity and then the rest. Just before this is done the external carotid should be identified where it emerges from behind the stylohyoid at its upper border and enters the deep surface of the gland. It is then ligated using an aneurysm needle and transected. This prevents troublesome hemorrhage from the maxillary artery as the medial pterygoid is sectioned. Strong downward traction will now permit separation of the insertion of the temporalis into the coronoid process. Any intact upper branches of the nerve are gathered upwards in a loop of tape and the specimen rotated outwards about the condyle to expose the lateral pterygoid muscle which is then divided under direct vision to complete the excision.

As hemostasis is completed the maxillary artery is sought and ligated. The facial nerve is repaired using the great auricular nerve as a graft as necessary and if possible part of temporalis is rotated down to cover the nerve graft. A bone graft of the mandible may be placed unless a postoperative course of radiotherapy is to be employed. Indeed, there is also some risk of failure even after preoperative radiotherapy. Bone grafting at a second operation carries an unacceptable risk to residual branches of the facial nerve and to any successful nerve graft. Recovery of function in the facial muscles is of more important than the continuity of the mandible. Where the ramus is not replaced by a bone graft the patient will be left with a deep depression in front of the ear but this can be covered by a suitable hair-style. There will also be a marked tendency for the mandible to swing towards the affected side and early training is necessary to overcome this. Even with a graft the patient must practice maintaining centric occlusion and control of the jaw with the remaining muscles as soon as the initial wound healing is complete.

From time to time it will be helpful to obtain wider clearance. Where the condyle is invaded the articular fossa and the eminentia can also be removed. The styloid process and the styloid muscles can be excised to increase the margin in the depths of the wound but this should be done after resection of the main mass. To attempt this before invites damage to the internal carotid artery and internal jugular vein before there is sufficient exposure for control of hemorrhage. While a further layer of tissue can be removed by this maneuver there are disadvantages. Once the styloid process and its muscles have gone the major vessels will be left uncovered at the bottom of a large potential dead space and protected only by a skin flap. Wound breakdown could lead to rupture of the internal carotid artery or the internal jugular vein. They should be covered by temporalis muscle to give them added protection.

Temporoparotidectomy[7]
Small scale resection of the external auditory canal may be included with the excision of the pinna and overlying skin of the parotid where these structures are involved. The deficiency may be made good with a deltopectoral or other suitable flap. Without great difficulty the mastoid process can also be detached. This may be done to uncover the trunk of the facial nerve sufficiently to make nerve suture and grafting possible. However, removing the bone of the external meatus and the mastoid process does little to improve the safety margin where bone has been invaded posteriorly.

The problems of treating a malignant neoplasm that is invading the temporal bone by radiotherapy are two-fold. First is to ensure an adequate margin within the irradiated volume whilst still avoiding high doses to the brain and second to treat effectively a tumor which is invading dense bone.

Consideration should be given to palliative radiation treatment alone, or pre- or postoperative radiotherapy and total parotidectomy, recognizing the limitations of these treatments, but being certain of a low operative mortality and relatively low morbidity. The alternative is a combination of preoperative radiotherapy and extensive radical surgery.

Excision of the temporal bone for carcinoma of the middle ear is a standard procedure, even though it is infrequently performed. Extension of a parotid neoplasm back into the temporal bone is therefore amenable to excision of the parotid gland, ramus of the mandible and temporomandibular joint together with the temporal bone. The operation carries considerable risk because of the need to section dense bone and separate it from the internal carotid artery, internal jugular vein and sigmoid, superior petrosal and inferior petrosal sinuses. Adequate cover needs to be provided for the dura as the wound is closed. The hypoglossal nerve is mobilized and anastomosed to peripheral branches of the facial nerve at the end of the operation.

Parotidectomy in continuity with neck dissection
Cervical lymph node metastases are not common in patients with cancer of the major salivary glands.[14] The reported overall incidence of clinical lymph node metastases is 16% for carcinomas of the parotid and 8% for submandibular and sublingual gland carcinomas.[15] Tumors of 4 cm or more in size have a 20% risk of occult metastasis to the cervical nodes as compared to 4% risk for smaller tumors. High grade tumors have a risk of occult metastasis to the cervical nodes of 49% as compared to 7% for intermediate and low grade tumors.[16] The management of neck in patients with salivary

194 Salivary gland pathologies

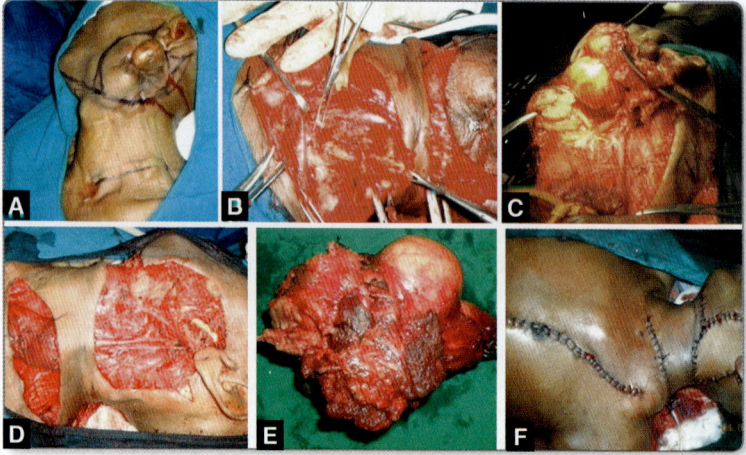

Figures 12.10A to F (A) McFee incision marked; (B) Radical neck dissection; (C) Total parotidectomyalong with facial nerve and overlying skin; (D) Postoperative defect; (E) Specimen; (F) Reconstruction with PMMC and closure

gland tumors is controversial. This is in part due to lack of consensus on the true rate of cervical metastasis which has been reported to be as high as 53% by Stennert E et al in 2003.[17] A radical neck dissection should be performed where the cervical lymph nodes are involved or where there is a mass at the lower pole of the parotid due to an aggressive tumor of such as size that invasion of the upper deep cervical nodes cannot be excluded. According to Armstrong JG et al, high grade tumors and advanced primary tumors of sizes more than 4 cm have a high rate of occult metastasis in the neck and hence treatment of the neck is indicated. However, small low-grade tumors have a low frequency of occult metastasis and routine elective neck dissection is not indicated.[15,16] Metastasis to the cervical nodes is not uncommon where there is recurrence after previous incomplete surgery, even where mucoepidermoid, acinic cell and adenoid cystic carcinomas are concerned and further operation should include a neck dissection. Consideration should be given to preoperative irradiation of the neck to a dose of 4000 to 5000 rads preoperatively (Henk 1976). Armstrong JG et al have suggested that combined neck dissection and neck irradiation may reduce neck recurrences and may be indicated if multiple neck nodes are palpable.[15]

Currently, it is thought that an elective neck dissection is seldom indicated in N0 neck cases in patients with malignant salivary gland tumors.[15,18] Elective neck dissection is appropriate only when the risk of occult metastasis is high. However, in cases wherein clinicopathologic

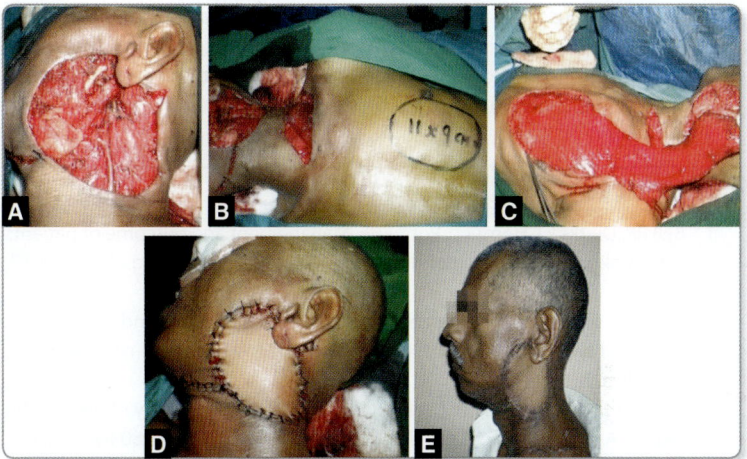

Figures 12.11A to E (A) Surgical defect ; (B) Marking of PMMC; (C) Harvesting of PMMC flap; (D) Closure; (E) Postoperative result

characteristics of the primary tumor are indicative of a high risk of occult metastasis, postoperative radiotherapy is indicated routinely for the primary tumor. In such cases, the need to address the neck during surgery is alleviated and post operative radiotherapy is sufficient to tackle the problem of occult metastasis.[14]

However, according to Bell et al, for any N-positive neck, regardless of histology or site comprehensive neck dissection should be carried out. In cases of N0 neck, clinically negative neck, selective neck dissection is advisable in patients with high grade tumors, locally advanced disease, facial nerve paralysis/weakness and advanced age. Management of neck in N0 cases of small, low grade tumors of minor salivary glands is unnecessary.[1]

The incidence of occult nodal metastasis is higher in patients with anaplastic, high-grade mucoepidermoid and salivary duct carcinoma and adenocarcinoma as compared to low-grade mucoepidermoid and acinic cell carcinoma.

Reconstruction[19]

This is required only if the skin has been resected and is usually provided by using a flap cover as only SSG is not conducive for successful nerve graft take. A free microvascular flap or a pedicled axial pattern flap can be used for reconstruction of the defect. Upper trapezius myocutaneous flap, pectoralis major myocutaneous (PMMC) flap, forehead flap, deltopectoral

(DP) flap, latissimus dorsi flap are examples of axial pattern pedicled flaps that can be used for reconstruction. Among microvascular flaps, free radial forearm flap, jejunal flap, dorsalis pedis flap, latissimus dorsi flap, composite groin flap can be used with satisfactory results.

References

1. Bell RB, Dierks EJ, Homer L, Potter BE. Management and outcome of patients with malignant salivary gland tumors. J Oral Maxillofac Surg. 2005;63:917-28.
2. Hanna EY, Suen JY. Malignant tumors of the salivary glands. Myers EN, Suen JY, Myers JN, Hanna EY, (eds). Cancer of the head and neck. 4th edn. Saunders. 21:pp.475-510.
3. Ferreria JL, Maurino N, Michael E, Ratinoff M, Rubio E. Surgery of the parotid region: A new approach. J Oral and Maxillofac Surg. 1990;48:803-7.
4. Farrior JB, Santini H. facial nerve identification in children. Otolaryngol Head Neck Surg. 1985;93:173.
5. Hanna EY, Lee S, Fan CY, Suen JY. Benign neoplasms of the salivary glands. Haughley BH, (Ed). Cummings Otolaryngology Head and Neck Surgery, 4th edn. Elsevier Mosby publication, 2005:60(2):1348-77.
6. Meningaud JP, Bertolus C, Bertrand JC. Parotidectomy: Assessment of A surgical technique including facelift incision and SMAS advancement. Journal of Cranio-maxillofacial Surg. 2006;34:34-7.
7. Shah JP. Color atlas of operative techniques in head and neck surgery. Wolfe Medical Publications, England, pp.117-33.
8. GYYU, DQ Ma, XB Liu, MY Zhang, Q Zhang. Local excision of the parotid gland in the treatment of Warthin's tumor. Br J Oral Maxillofac Surg. 1988;36:186-9.
9. Johns M, Nachlas N. Salivary gland tumors Paperella, Shumrick, Gluckman, Meyerhoff editors. Otolaryngology, 3rd edn. WB Saunders Company, Philadelphia. 1991;20(3):2099-127.
10. Kun Z, Dao-Yi Q, Li-Min W. Functional superficial parotidectomy. J Oral Maxillofac Surg. 1994;52:1038-41.
11. Nikolaos Papadogeorgakis, Chris A. Skouteris, Anastassios I. Mylonas, Angelos P, Angelopoulos. Superficial parotidectomy: technical modifications based on tumor characteristics. J Cranio Maxillofacs Surg. 2004;32:350-3.
12. Yamashita T, Tomoda K, Kumazawa T. The usefulness of partial parotidectomy for benign parotid gland tumors. Acta Otolaryngol. 1993;500:113-6.
13. Oslen KD. Intraoral salivary gland tumor removal. Section I Head and Neck (Eds). Bailey BJ. Atlas of head and neck surgery–Otolaryngology, 2nd edn. Bailey BJ, Calhoun KH, Friedman NR, Newlands SD, Vrabec JT. Eds. Lippincott Williams and Wilkins. Philadelphia. pp. 6-7.
14. Medina JE. Neck dissection in the treatment of cancer of major salivary glands. Otolaryngologic clinics of North America. 1998;31(5):815-22.

15. Armstrong JG, Harrison LB, Thaler HT, Friedlander-Klar H, Fass DE, Zelefsky MJ, et al. The indications for elective treatment of the neck in cancer of the major salivary glands. Cancer. 1992;69:615-9.
16. Hanna EY, Suen JY. The Parotid Neoplasm. Pensak ML (Ed). Controversies in Otolaryngology. Publication Thieme. Newyork. 2001;66(22):348-54.
17. Bell RB, Dierks EJ, Homer L, Potter BE. Management and outcome of patients with malignant salivary gland tumors. J Oral Maxillofac Surg. 2005;63:917-28.
18. Frankenthaler RA, Byers RM, Luna MA, et al. Predicting occult lymph node metastasis in parotid cancer. Arch Otolaryngol Head and Neck Surg. 1993;119:517-20.
19. McGregor IA, McGregor FM. Cancer of the face and mouth. Salivary Tumors. Churchill Livingstone, New York. 1986;25:569-606.

Surgical management of submandibular and sublingual neoplasms

chapter 13

Surgical management of cancer of the submandibular salivary gland depends on the extent of the tumor. Small tumors confined to the gland itself are treated by resection of the submandibular gland. Tumors spreading beyond the confines of the gland to invade surrounding structures are treated with a wider en bloc excision. This may require removal of the contents of the submandibular triangle; resection of the floor of the mouth and the mylohyoid and digastric muscles; or marginal or segmental mandibulectomy, depending on the extent of the tumor. Special attention should be given to the lingual, hypoglossal, mylohyoid and marginal mandibular nerves because these may be involved through perineural spread of tumor. Thickening and nodularity of these nerves may indicate perineural involvement; in such cases, histologic confirmation by frozen section may be useful in both establishing nerve invasion and obtaining negative surgical margins.[1,2]

Incision for access to submandibular gland

The incision line runs within a skin crease in the neck at least 3 cm below the lower border of the mandible in order to avoid risk of damaging the mandibular branch of the facial nerve as it loops down below the lower border of the mandible **(Figure 13.1)**. It should be approximately 7 cm long.

The lower the incision within the neck, the better the post-operative cosmetic result, but incisions lower than 3 cm make the operation slightly more difficult as the operator must dissect upwards to reach the submandibular triangle.

Incision for excision of sublingual gland

For simple excision of the sublingual gland, a linear incision is made in the floor of the mouth parallel to and just lateral to the submandibular duct, with care taken not to extend the incision more posteriorly than the first molar tooth so as to avoid damage to the lingual nerve. When sublingual gland excision is necessary for a tumor, it should be removed with a wide margin including a rim resection of the mandible.

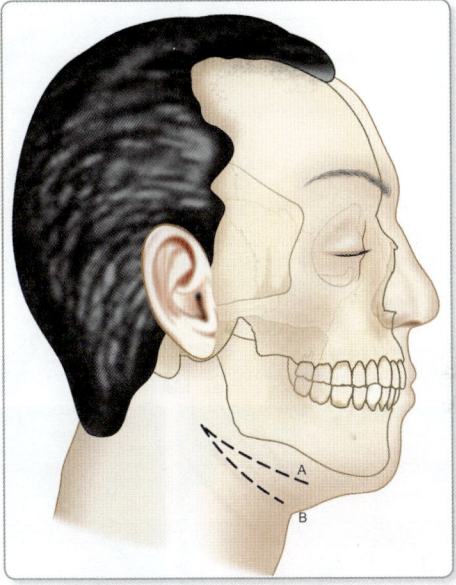

Figure 13.1 Submandibular incision

Extra capsular excision of the submandibular salivary gland[3]

There is a higher incidence of recurrence for the submandibular gland than for the parotid after excision of slow growing neoplasms including pleomorphic adenoma. This should not be so because the surgical procedure is less difficult. The surgical procedure is carried out under general anesthesia unless the patient's medical status contraindicates the same. A curvilinear incision is placed 2–3 cm below the inferior border of the mandible and should be hidden in a skin crease if possible. The skin incision is injected with lignocaine with adrenaline solution for hemostasis. The anesthetist should avoid the use of paralyzing agents if possible. The incision is approximately 5–7 cm in length and is carried down through the subcutaneous fat and platysma. The capsule of the gland and surrounding soft tissue must be left intact over the gland when the surgical procedure is being carried out for a neoplastic growth. The gland is removed together with its investing fascia, which is separated from the anterior and posterior bellies of the digastric and the stylohyoid muscle. This technique endangers the marginal mandibular nerve and hence the facial artery and vein are

200 Salivary gland pathologies

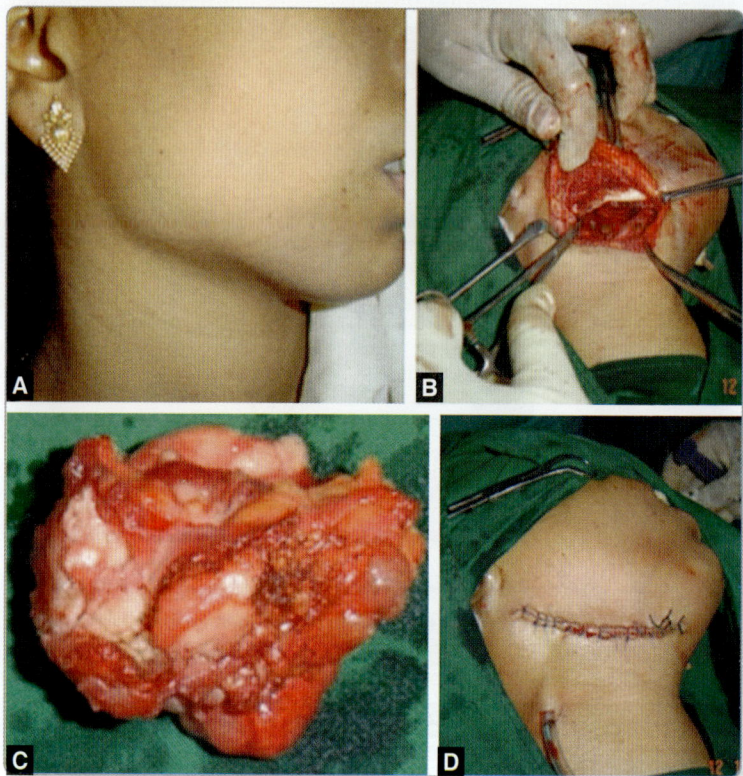

Figures 13.2A to D (A) Tumor involving submandibular gland; (B) Tumor excised through submandibular incision; (C) Specimen; (D) Closure

identified early in their course as close to the gland as possible and after transection should be elevated superiorly to identify and reflect the marginal mandibular nerve from the field. The marginal mandibular branch of the facial nerve is isolated and preserved and then the fascia is divided at the lower border of the mandible. The facial artery is again transected posterolaterally near its origin from the carotid artery.

Anteriorly the gland needs to be separated from the mylohyoid muscle but if necessary some muscle can be included in the specimen. As the superficial part of the gland is dissected from the muscle, posterolateral border is encountered. Three vital structures are identified here viz. lingual nerve, hypoglossal nerve and Wharton's duct. The free edge of the mylohyoid is retracted medially. The lingual nerve shares the same facial

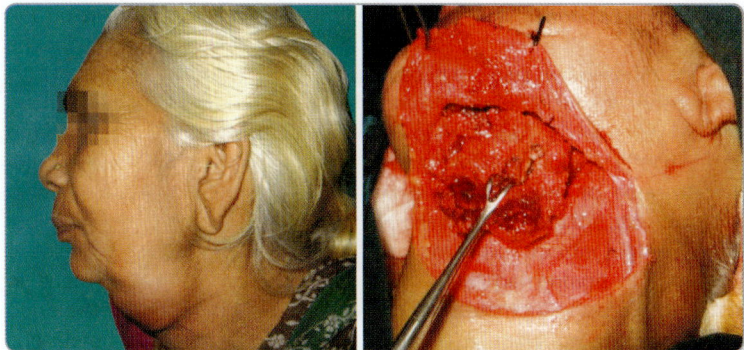

Figure 13.3 Submandibular gland tumor excision through submandibular incision

sheath as the gland at the upper pole. This attachment of the lingual nerve to the gland represents its parasympathetic supply. The Wharton's duct is inferior to lingual nerve and is often surrounded by sublingual glands. As fascia and gland are mobilized upwards from the surface of the hyoglossus the hypoglossal nerve is identified more inferiorly. It is accompanied by ranine vein which may aid in its identification. In addition veni comitans accompany the nerve and are inevitably damaged and hemostasis must be affected with care to avoid damage to the nerve. Both the nerve and the accompanying vein emerge from beneath the digastric and pass anterosuperiorly into the tongue. Posteriorly the angular tract of fascia has to be cut with scissors to allow the gland in its fascial envelope to be drawn down. This step is the most difficult because it is important not to grasp the gland with instruments, particularly tissue forceps lest the tumor be ruptured. Where necessary the upper pole may be mobilized via the mouth. An assistant can then depress the gland towards the submandibular wound to enable the operation to be concluded.

The duct and the branch of the lingual nerve supplying the submandibular gland are ligated and transected. The duct is divided close behind the papilla. During excision for inflamma-tory disease the nerve is always separated from the gland with knife or scissors. However if the nerve appears to be involved in a tumor it is sectioned in front of and behind the gland and the cut ends sutured. Should a greater margin of tissue than the immediate capsule be required laterally, then the periosteum of the mandible is divided along the lower border and stripped up from the submandibular fossa. It must be divided at the level of the mylohyoid line so that the lingual nerve can be found and freed as described above. The wound is closed in layers with drainage in the usual way.

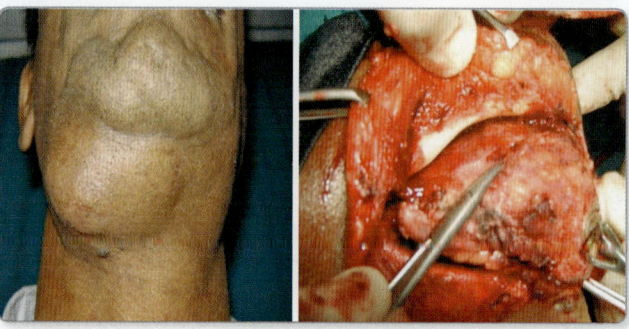

Figure 13.4 Showing adenoid cystic carcinoma involving the sublingual salivary gland

Radical excision of neoplasms of the submandibular or sublingual salivary gland[3]

Excision of a frankly malignant, invasive neoplasm of the submandibular or sublingual salivary gland will include the tongue on that side, the floor of the mouth and the mandible together with a radical neck dissection if palpable nodes are present.

References

1. Hanna EY, Suen JY. Malignant tumors of the salivary glands. Myers EN, Suen JY, Myers JN, Hanna EY, editors. Cancer of the head and neck. 4th ed. Saunders. 21.pp.475-510.
2. Weber RS, Byers RM, Petit B, et al. Submandibular gland tumors. Adverse histologic factors and therapeutic implications. Arch Otolaryngol Head Neck Surg. 1990;116:1055-60.
3. Seward GR. Nodular enlargement of a salivary gland. Moore, Editor. Surgery of the Mouth and Jaws. Blackwell Scientific Publication. London. 1985; 38:676-99.

Surgical management of minor salivary gland neoplasms

chapter 14

Surgical resection of cancer of the minor salivary gland depends on the site of origin and extent of disease. In the oral cavity, this may require only a wide local excision of localized low-grade tumors. Larger and/or high-grade tumors may require more radical excision, including marginal or segmental mandibulectomy and/or partial or total resection of the hard or soft palate. Salivary gland cancers involving the sinonasal tract is usually of high grade and presents at an advanced stage. Surgical resection may require partial or total maxillectomy, infratemporal fossa dissection, and/or anterior craniofacial resection. Palatal defects resulting from these resections are best managed by prosthetic rehabilitation. The branches of the second (V2) and third (V3) divisions of the trigeminal nerve are at high risk for perineural spread of minor salivary gland malignancy. These nerves may provide an avenue for early skull base invasion. Resection of the cranial base may be required in some cases to eradicate the tumor and obtain negative surgical margins.[1]

Malignant minor salivary gland neoplasms are generally treated by composite resection via transoral or transfacial approaches depending on site, size and tumor histology.

Excision of palatal pleomorphic adenomas[2]

Small palatal pleomorphic adenomas usually cause pressure resorption of the palate but do not invade the bone. A disc of palatal mucosa is outlined well clear of the visible swelling because the tumor is flattened owing to the toughness of the palatal tissues. The incision is deepened to bone and the specimen reflected off the hard palate, taking care to include the periosteum. Where it overlies the soft palate, scissors are used to cut the tissues and

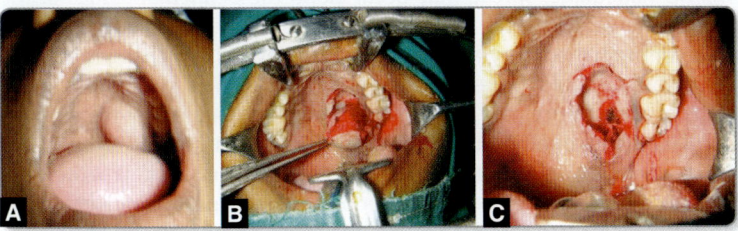

Figures 14.1A to C (A) Pleomorphic adenoma of palate; (B) Excision of tumor; (C) Surgical defect

ensure a margin around the tumor. In general the plane of dissection can be carried back from the palate over the surface of the tendon of tensor palati. The neoplasm frequently sits over the greater palatine foramen and the periosteum is freed here until the lesion can be drawn down and the vessels and nerve above the tumor seen. The neurovascular bundle is clamped with artery forceps, sectioned and the cut end coagulated by diathermy before it is released. This is necessary to affect hemostasis before the vessels retract up the canal.

Interrupted silk sutures are tied by one end around the periphery of the wound and a pack of ribbon gauze soaked in Whitehead's varnish inserted. The sutures are tied together in a spider's web to retain the pack. Where circumscribing the tumor means the removal of the full thickness of the soft palate the defect may be repaired by an island flap, based on the opposite greater palatine artery, as described by Worthington (1974).

Excision of palatal mucoepidermoid carcinoma[2]

The margin to be taken around the tumor will depend upon its aggressiveness. Low-grade muco-epidermoid carcinomas may be treated by the excision of a full thickness disc of palate, including palatal and alveolar bone. Nasal and oral mucous membranes are sewn together around the defect in the soft palate and a gutta percha obturator fitted. It is not necessary to cover this with a skin graft unless the operation extends on to the lateral surface of the maxilla. The acrylic palate supporting the obturator is retained with cribs on the natural teeth if possible or by circum-zygomatic wires if the patient is edentulous. As these neoplasms may be very slow growing a considerable time may elapse before a recurrence is detected, so that surgical repair of the defect is contraindicated until at least five years after treatment. Once the palate has been repaired there will be little chance of spotting a recurrence until it is quite large and it could involve the orbit or base of the skull.

Excision of palatal adenoid cystic carcinoma[2]

The danger with these neoplasms is the risk that the surgical margin will be inadequate. Spread may occur along the perineural tissues of the palatine nerves taking the tumor up to the base of the skull. It may also take place through medullary alveolar bone well beyond any changes seen on radiographs. Should the lesion not be eradicated at the first attempt the first signs of a recurrence may be pain in the pharynx, paralysis of the external occular muscles or other signs indicative of intracranial spread.

A combination of surgery and radiotherapy is best. Whether the latter is given by external beam preoperatively or postoperatively, or by postoperative intracavity irradiation, will depend upon the site and size of the neoplasm. Surgical excision should be generous. Hemimaxillectomy

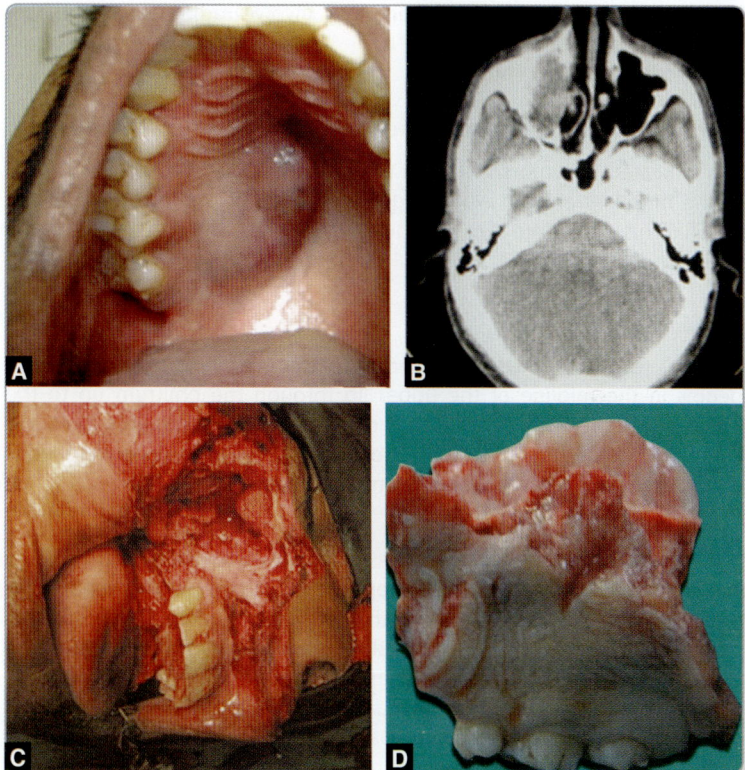

Figures 14.2A to D (A) Tumor of palatal minor salivary gland; (B) CT scan showing involvement of maxillary sinus; (C) Subtotal maxillectomy and post-surgical defect; (D) Specimen

including the orbital floor is a minimum unless there is very good evidence that less will be sufficient. Where the soft palate and pterygoid region is involved, extended maxillectomy approach is essential to ensure adequate excision under direct vision.

Excision of neoplasms of cheek and lips[2]

Slow growing lumps may be removed with a margin of normal adjacent tissue, using scissors to effect the dissection. With discretion a primary excision can be used, but if there is any doubt in the mind of the operator a biopsy should be taken first. Re-operation following incomplete extirpation could mean the unnecessary sacrifice of tissue to ensure an adequate margin on the second occasion. Clinically aggressive neoplasms must be biopsied, since adequate treatment may involve radiotherapy and full-thickness excision and repair.

Partial maxillectomy[3]

It is indicated in tumors involving the upper gingiva, hard palate or floor of the maxillary antrum which requires removal of the lower half of the maxilla. This procedure is carried out under general anesthesia and under oro-tracheal intubation.

Incision

Weber – Fergusson incision is used for partial maxillectomy. The incision begins in the midline of the upper lip through the philtrum up to the collumella of the nasal cavity. Here it curves around the nasal vestibule and ala of the nostril up to the naso – labial crease and then along naso-labial crease to the region of the medial canthus of the eye.

Surgical procedure

The cheek flap is raised. When the upper lip is cut, bleeding is encountered from the superior labial artery, which needs to be ligated. The next cut is given at the upper gingivobuccal sulcus mucosa and full thickness flap is elevated. Infraorbital nerve and its entry into soft tissues, is exposed. It is preserved only if lower half of the maxilla is to be resected.

The cheek flap is elevated as far back as posterolateral surface of maxilla exposing undersurface of zygoma to gain access to pterygomaxillary fissure. Entry is made in to the nasal cavity by dividing soft tissues along ala of nose until mucosa of lateral wall of nasal cavity is completely divided. Then, ala of nostril is retracted medially and rest of the mucosa of the floor of the nasal cavity up to nasal bone is incised. This provides a satisfactory exposure.

The mouth is opened wide with a mouth gag to provide adequate exposure of the alveolar process and hard palate. Then the maxillary antrum is entered with a drill bit and drill midway between infraorbital foramen and alveolar process. The cut is then extended anteriorly and posteriorly to create a line of transection through the anterior wall of the maxillary sinus to allow division of the lower half of the maxilla. The cut is carried anteriorly through the nasal process and posteriorly up to zygomatic process of the maxilla and around the posterolateral surface of the maxilla. A tooth is extracted at the proposed line of transection of alveolar process. The transverse and vertical cuts are connected.

The palatal mucosa is then incised around the tumor with an adequate and satisfactory margin in all directions. Posteriorly the incision begins at maxillary tubercle and then curves medially and to the anterior aspect of the tumor with adequate clearance. Mucosal incision is then deepened up to bone throughout the length. Hard palate is divided through the line of mucosal incision with rotory instruments or with right angled or sagittal saw. After all bony cuts are made; osteotome is used to connect the fracture lines permitting the specimen to be rocked over soft tissue attachments. With the help of cautery or heavy mayo scissors, the posterior soft tissue attachments, i.e. pterygoid muscles are divided and surgical specimen of lower half of maxilla is delivered.

This step of removal of the surgical specimen should be carried out as fast as possible because there is occurrence of brisk bleeding from palatine vessels and branches of internal maxillary artery coming from the posterior wall and pterygoid fossa in to the maxilla as well as sphenopalatine artery and small arteries of the soft palate, which can be controlled, only after surgical specimen is removed. Bleeding from the internal maxillary artery is controlled by ligation and that from the sphenopalatine artery by electrocoagulation. Maxillary sinus mucosa can be seen, which if inflamed, is curetted out and sent for histopathological examination. The bony margins are smoothened. The cut edges of mucosa of posterior and anterior wall of soft palate is sutured with catgut. The raw surfaces of the oral mucosa and bone may be covered with split thickness skin graft. The antral defect is packed with iodoform guaze. Palatal obturator must be placed in the defect and skin sutured in two layers.

Total maxillectomy

A total maxillectomy becomes necessary when the tumor fills up the entire maxillary antrum. The surgical exposure for total maxillectomy is similar to partial maxillectomy, only difference being that total maxillectomy requires a much wider exposure.

Incision

A modified Weber-Fergusson incision is used for total maxillectomy. In this in addition to the original incision, an extension, called as Diffenbach extension is employed along tarsal margin of lower eyelid up to the lateral canthus of the eye. This provides adequate exposure of zygomatic process of maxilla as well as region of pterygomaxillary fissure and is hence used for total maxillectomy.

Surgical procedure

The upper cheek flap is elevated as usual with a mucosal incision in the upper gingivobuccal sulcus all the way up to the maxillary tubercle posteriorly. It may have to be extended to reach the retromolar trigone for additional exposure. The lateral skin incision is placed as close to the eyelashes as possible to avoid an unsightly scar and edematous lower eyelid. While raising the flap, care should be exercised at the lower eyelid to avoid skin perforation, because there is lack of subcutaneous tissue between the orbicularis oculi muscle and overlying skin. The infraorbital nerve is divided at its exit from the infraorbital foramen.

The cheek flap, elevated in its entirety, exposes the anterior and anterolateral wall of the maxilla, and can be rapidly elevated with minimal blood loss using electrocautery. Entry into the nasal cavity is obtained by retracting the ala of the nose anteriorly and dividing the soft tissue attachments on the nasal process of the maxilla to provide access. Then the cut edge of the skin incision is retracted medially, elevating the skin over the nose and exposing the nasal bone. Then, using a power saw the nasal process of the maxilla is divided, and a periosteal elevator is used to elevate the periosteum of the orbit from its bony floor. This elevation extends from the medial cut on the maxilla up to the transection margin of the zygomatic process laterally, and is taken as far back as possible on its floor to maintain the orbital surface of the maxilla intact for monobloc resection of the surgical specimen. No attempt is made to elevate the periosteum from the medial and the lateral walls of the orbit since bony attachment of the periosteum on these walls is necessary to prevent inferior displacement of the globe postoperatively. A power saw is used to divide the zygomatic process of the maxilla at the level required depending upon the anatomical location of the primary tumor. In order to expose this, extreme lateral retraction of the cheek flap with a rake retractor is necessary. Zygomatic process of the maxilla is a sturdy segment of solid bone that requires a deep, bony cut to obtain satisfactory mobilization of the specimen. Complete division of the zygomatic process may require the use of an osteotome since using a power saw in the deeper plane could traumatize the orbital contents or, laterally, the soft tissues of the infratemporal fossa. After this procedure, superior mobilization of the surgical specimen is almost complete. Brisk bleeding is encountered from the cut edges of the zygoma. Electrocautery is then used to divide the soft tissues over the premaxilla in the midline anteriorly giving adequate exposure of the medial margin of the surgical specimen.

The oral cavity is now opened wide using a retractor. An incision is made in the midline of the mucosa of the hard palate up to the junction of the hard and soft palate posteriorly, and extended deeply through the mucoperiosteum up to the bone. Then a lateral mucosal incision is made along the posterior edge of the hard palate at the junction of the hard and soft palate up to the maxillary tubercle, and taken deeply through the musculature of the soft palate, partly to provide soft tissue mobilization posteromedially. The midline of the hard palate is then divided through the floor of the nasal cavity up to the junction of the hard and soft palate using a power saw. The medial mobilization of the surgical specimen by fracturing the hard palate can also be accomplished by using a straight osteotome since the fracture is linear. Bleeding from cut edges of the bone is brisk and immediate hemostasis is not satisfactory, so speed is of utmost importance during this phase of the operation until the surgical specimen is removed.

The cheek flap is now retracted laterally as far as possible to provide exposure and access to the posterior wall of the maxilla and the pterygomaxillary fissure. The soft tissue attachments in this area, as well as the presence of the buccal fat pad, makes visualization of this area difficult but the pterygomaxillary fissure and the tuberosity of the maxilla can easily be palpated. A curved osteotome is then used to separate the specimen through the pterygomaxillary fissure. The maxilla is separated from the pterygoid plates by placing the curved osteotome in the fissure; and applying gentle strokes with a mallet. This mobilization again results in brisk hemorrhage from branches of the internal maxillary artery. Once bony separation in this area is achieved, this specimen can be rocked by digital maneuvers. Medial and lateral soft tissue attachments should be divided with the help of electrocautery or heavy, curved Mayo scissors; the final separation of the orbital surface of the maxilla is achieved using Mayo scissors. As the specimen is rocked, soft tissue attachments come into view and they should be divided under direct vision leading to final delivery of the specimen. Extreme care and attention should be paid to gentle handling and division of the soft tissues during this phase of the operation, as rough handling may result in fracture of the specimen and spillage of the tumor.

Once the surgical specimen is removed, several bleeding points can be identified, most of which are from branches of the internal maxillary and the sphenopalatine artery. Following adequate hemostasis, the surgical defect is irrigated with saline. The surgical defect is also inspected to assure the adequacy of surgical resection, and frozen sections from soft tissue margins can be obtained at this time. All sharp, bony spicules are smoothed out with a burr. Every attempt should be made to preserve the integrity of the orbital periosteum since any breech in its wall will cause prolapse of periorbital fat.

A split-thickness skin graft is obtained and applied beginning at the superolateral aspect of the surgical defect, the orbital periosteum and the soft tissues in the pterygoid fossa. The undersurface of the cheek flap is also covered with a skin graft, which is usually secured with interrupted 3-0 chromic catgut sutures. A rim of soft tissues is spared at the medial edge of the cheek flap for subcutaneous sutures. Once the skin graft is sutured in position, it is molded into the surgical defect covering all its crevices and corners using xeroform gauze packing, which is placed digitally and under moderate pressure to stretch the skin graft and retain it in position. The previously fabricated immediate dental obturator is now applied to replace the resected portion of the hard palate. If the patient has teeth remaining, the dental obturator is wired to them. But if the patient is edentulous, holes are drilled into the contralateral alveolar process through which wires are

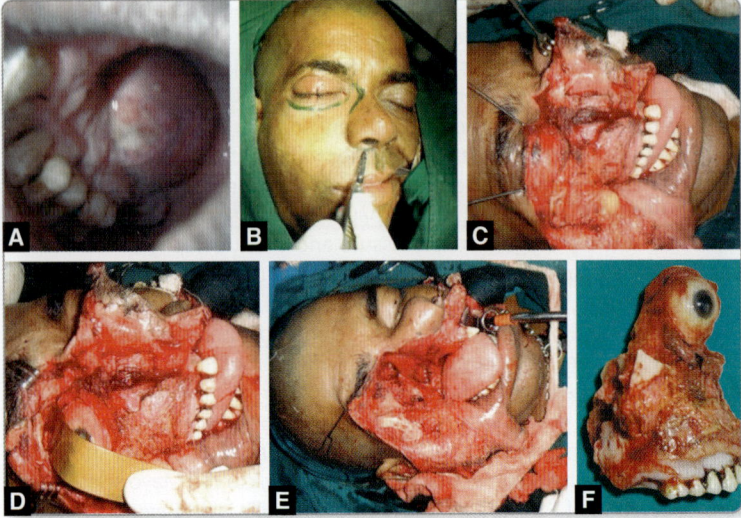

Figures 14.3A to F (A) Intraoral lesion; (B) Weber-Fergusson incision; (C) Flap elevated; (D) Orbital periosteum raised; (E) Surgical defect; (F) Specimen

passed for retention of the dental obturator. The latter supports the packing and restores the continuity of the roof of the mouth to allow satisfactory swallowing in the immediate postoperative period. The skin incision is next closed as usual in two layers, paying special attention to detail in closure of the lateral extension. An absorbable, continuous subcuticular suture extending from the medial to the lateral canthus is preferred since it avoids any irritation of the eye and provides a very satisfactory approximation of the skin edges. No dressings are necessary. Bacitracin skin ointment is applied to the suture line.

Extended maxillectomy

Extended maxillectomies are indicated when the extent of disease is beyond the confines of the maxilla. It may involve the inclusion of additional structures into the specimen such as; eye exenteration, obase of the skull.

Postoperative care

Postoperative care for the partial maxillectomy as well as total maxillectomy patient is similar. Extraoral and intraoral wound care is performed. Warm compresses are placed over cheek occasionally to control swelling and inflammation. Patients are encouraged and trained to perform frequent oral irrigation particularly after each meal, and exercises of the jaw to prevent trismus and relieve pain due to fibrosis. However, in total maxillectomy, minor bleeding from the raw areas and granulation tissue in the pterygoid fossa is common and may require cauterization with silver nitrate; oral exercises are mandatory for several months to prevent trismus; fabrication of the definitive dental obturator should take into consideration obliteration of the air space in the surgical defect to restore satisfactory quality of voice. This is achieved by bolus extension of the dental obturator.

References

1. Hanna EY, Suen JY. Malignant tumors of the salivary glands. Myers EN, Suen JY, Myers JN, Hanna EY, (Eds). Cancer of the head and neck, 4th edn. Saunders. 21.pp.475-510.
2. Hanna EY, Suen JY. The Parotid Neoplasm. Controversies in Otolaryngology. Pensak ML (Ed). Publication Thieme. Newyork. 2001;66(22)348-54.
3. Shah JP. Color atlas of Operative techniques in Head and Neck Surgery. Wolfe Medical Publications, England. pp.117-33.

Complications of salivary gland surgery

chapter 15

Since all surgical procedures are not without complications, so salivary gland tumor surgeries too can land up in complications. In general the complications that can be faced are as follows:

Hematoma

The dead space that is created due to removal of part or whole of the salivary gland fills up with blood unless measures are taken to prevent this eventuality. Most important precaution to avoid this complication is achieving good hemostasis before wound closure. In addition provision of adequate drainage by using drains must be carried out. In case a rubber corrugated drain is placed then wide drain of 4–5 corrugations must be used and a pressure dressing must be placed over the operated site to obliterate any potential space that is created due to surgery. An alternative is to use a suction drain of a larger diameter if feasible. In case of parotid surgeries, care should be taken to place the tube deep to digastric muscle to avoid the sucking of the facial nerve. A pressure dressing can be given in addition.

In case a hematoma develops, then care should be taken to avoid infection by prescribing high antibiotics to the patient. The hematoma can be aspirated or sucked under aseptic precautions. However, it may not be completely effective. Eventually a hematoma will resolve without getting infected.[1]

Trismus

Trismus after parotidectomy is commonly seen post-op complication. It is probably related to masseter muscle spasm or inflammatory changes in the TMJ capsule secondary to trauma. This condition is self limiting and hence premature use of mouth gags to forcefully open the jaws should be avoided because of the tremendous pain associated with this condition. In fact it could lead to aggravation of the pain symptoms and increased trismus. Most of the cases resolve spontaneously without any active intervention. However, in long standing cases use of intra-articular injections of hydrocortisone and long acting local anesthetics in the TMJ might prove to be beneficial.[1]

Salivary fistula

It is a quite uncommon phenomenon. Its likely cause is discontinuity between the residual salivary gland parenchyma and the salivary duct. However, since after every parotidectomy it doesn't form and hence this is not the likely cause.[1] It usually presents as a clear sialorrhea from the wound or a fluid collection under the skin flaps.[2] It could be due to an over secretion of saliva leading to seepage of saliva out of the wound.[1]

In majority of cases the problem is self limiting. Management includes repeated aspiration, pressure dressings, wound care and patience. In addition, an antisialogogue medication (glycopyrolate) may be prescribed to decrease the amount of salivary secretion.[1,2]

Facial nerve paresis or paralysis

Facial nerve dysfunction may result from traction injury to the facial nerve during dissection. Until the anatomic integrity of the nerve is preserved, traction results in neuropraxia. In this case, complete recovery of nerve function within few months is anticipated. It may range from minimal partial weakness of either of the branches to complete paralysis of the entire nerve. Mehle et al observed 46% temporary dysfunction and only 4% permanent dysfunction in patients who underwent parotid surgery.[3] Similarly, in submandibular or sublingual gland surgery, temporary or permanent injury to marginal mandibular branch of facial nerve can occur. Nerve injury can be reduced by careful handling of the nerve. Overzealous traction should be avoided. In case the nerve is transected it should be followed by immediate nerve grafting repair. In case of complete facial paralysis, care should be taken to avoid exposure keratitis of the eye by use of artificial tears. A temporary tarsoraphy can also be performed.

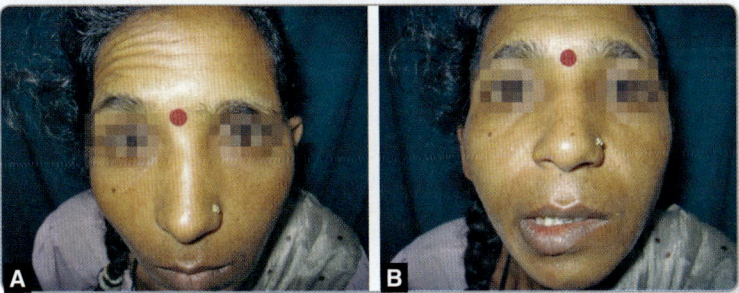

Figures 15.1A and B (A) Loss of wrinkling of forehead; (B) Deviation of mouth to opposite side

Auriculotemporal syndrome of frey

About one in ten patients undergoing parotid surgery suffer from gustatory sweating. It manifests as flushing and sweating of the skin of upper cheek, temporal region, and forehead coincident with eating, smelling of food.[4] The true incidence is unknown, but is estimated to be between 35% and 60%.[2]

The pathophysiology of this complication is as follows. Following damage to the auriculotemporal nerve or to communi-cating branches to the facial nerve, secretomotor parasympathetic nerves from the otic ganglion and also sympathetic fibers to the sweat glands traveling in the same nerve are divided. Following regeneration, fibers from otic ganglion come to supply the sweat glands. Thus there is cross-reinnervation between the postganglionic secretomotor parasympathetic fibers to parotid gland and postganglionic sympathetic fibers to the sweat glands of skin.[2]

Diagnosis is based on patient's symptoms. An objective method of confirming diagnosis is by Minor's starch-iodine test. This involves painting the involved side of face and neck with iodine solution which is allowed to dry. Starch powder is dusted over the area. Patient is asked to chew on a sialogogue for several minutes. The appearance of dark blue spots confirms the diagnosis.[2]

If symptoms are bothersome, simple treatment of antiperspirant application can be done. 1% local application of glycopyrrolate is effective.[2] Historically, tympanic neurectomy has been previously advocated by Golding-Wood, 1962, without much success. Shaheen OH has even attempted solving this problem by sectioning auriculotemporal nerve, but without any relief. Coldwater KB, 1954 has been suggested that secretomotor fibers which cause the sweating are located in the facial nerve and are relayed to the adjacent cutaneous nerves by anastomotic branches.[1]

Wallis KA et al have tried lifting the preauricular skin away from underlying soft tissues to interrupt nerve endings or excised parotid skin and used grafts or local transposition flaps without much relief. They have even tried using Fascia lata interpositioning with more success. Kornblut AD et al, 1974, have tried use of interpositioning of muscle between skin and remaining parotid tissue without much benefit.[1]

The only effective cure is to divide the parasympathetic fibers from the glossopharyngeal nerve either during their intracranial course in the lesser superficial petrosal nerve or in the tympanic and hypotympanic branches of glossopharyngeal nerve where they lie behind the round window on inner aspect of middle ear.[4] More recently, Kuttner C et al, 2001 have suggested intracutaneous injection of Botulinum toxin A as an effective treatment.[2]

Sensory abnormalities associated with greater auricular nerve sacrifice

The greater auricular nerve is frequently divided during parotidectomy. This results in a sensory deficit in the dermatomal distribution of the nerve which includes lower-third of pinna including earlobe as well as adjacent preauricular and postauricular skin. However, it has been shown that this does not significantly affect the quality of life of the postoperative patient.

References

1. Problems in H & N surgery.
2. Hanna EY, Suen JY. Malignant tumors of the salivary glands. Myers EN, Suen JY, Myers JN, Hanna EY, editors. Cancer of the head and neck. 4th ed. Saunders. 21.pp.475-510.
3. Mehle ME, Kraus DH, Wood BG, et al. Facial nerve morbidity following parotid surgery for benign disease: The Cleaveland clinic Foundation experience. Laryngoscope. 1993;103:386-8.
4. Seward GR. Nodular enlargement of a salivary gland. Moore, Editor. Surgery of the Mouth and Jaws. Blackwell Scientific Publication. London. 1985;38:676-99.

Chemotherapy and radiotherapy

chapter 16

Traditionally salivary gland tumors were considered to be radioresistant, however management of malignant salivary gland neoplasms has changed in recent years. Historically salivary gland tumors have been considered resistant to low LET radiation (Linear energy transfer radiation), however information that has been accumulated over a period of years suggests that postoperative photon irradiation improves local control rates in patients with high risk of residual microscopic disease.[1] Refined imaging technology, the use of external beam radiation, neutron beam therapy and chemotherapy has altered management strategies for patients with salivary gland malignancies during the last two decades. Postoperative radiotherapy has shown to improve locoregional control for patients with advanced-stage gland cancer. Reports suggest that use of adjuvant radiotherapy in conjunction with surgery is superior to surgery alone in treatment of high-grade and/or advanced cancers of the parotid gland.[2,3,4]

Adenoid cystic carcinoma has been reported to be the most consistent radioresponsive tumor type.[5] Theriault and Fitzpatrick have reported that out of 271 parotid carcinomas, patients treated with combined therapy had a 10 year relapse free rate of 62% as compared to 22% for those treated by surgery alone.[2]

Bell et al recommend adjuvant radiotherapy of up to 6300 cGy delivered to the primary tumor site and high-risk lymph nodes. In cases of adenoid cystic carcinoma wherein there is perineural spread radiotherapy should also be directed along the path of the cranial nerve at risk for involvement.[3] Hanna E et al have recommended a postoperative radiation dose of 60 Gy (50–75 Gy) in 30 fractions to the operative bed. In cases of named nerve invasion the path of the nerve should be treated electively up to its ganglion.[6]

Wide-field radiation therapy to the parotid glands may result in significant complications, including severe xerostomia, sensorineural hearing loss, osteoradionecrosis of the temporal bone and radiation injury to the temporal lobe. Recent advances in the delivery of radiation therapy including three-dimensional conformal radiotherapy (3DCRT) and intensity-modulated radiotherapy (IMRT) have led to better tumor dosimetry and relative sparing of surrounding normal structures such as the oral cavity, cochlea and brain.[6]

The addition of adjuvant radiotherapy should not be considered as an adequate substitute for clear surgical margins. However in cases where it is not possible to achieve clear surgical margins, postoperative radiotherapy enhances local control.[2]

Neutron beam therapy was introduced in the past two decades and has been shown to improve locoregional control rates (67%) for advanced stage tumors in both Europe and United States of America.[3]

Fractionated neutron irradiation has high relative biologic effectiveness in many salivary gland histologic types as compared to conventional radiation. Unlike low LET radiation neutrons interact with the atomic nuclei of cells and produce densely ionizing protons which transfer high amounts of energy to the tumor and inflict significant percentage of single-hit double-stranded DNA damage. This type of radiation-induced damage is considered lethal and irreparable. By contrast, LET radiation is more sparsely ionizing and has a higher percentage of single-stranded DNA damage. Hence the capacity of potentially lethal repair in a neoplasm is reduced substantially in tumors irradiated with neutrons as compared with those treated with low LET radiation. Photon radiation causes most of the damage through generation of free radicals. This process depends biochemically on presence of oxygen in the cell. By contrast, neutrons depend less on oxygen to act as a mediator and have a greater tendency to cause damage through a direct interaction with tumor cells.[1]

2-year follow-up	Neutron therapy (%)	Photon Therapy (%)
Initial complete response	85	33
Locoregional control	67	17
2-year survival	62	25

(Data from Griffin TW, Pajak TF, Laramore GE et al. Neutron vs photon irradiation of inoperable salivary gland tumors: Results of an RTOG-MRC cooperative randomized study. Int J Radiation Oncol Biol Phys 15:1085-90. 1988)[6]

In cases of inoperable tumors, fast-neutron radiation therapy provides higher rates of locoregional control of the unresectable salivary gland cancer as compared to photon or electron radiation therapy.[1,2,7] According to a study by Laramore et al, conventional photon irradiation in the setting of locally advanced disease, recurrent disease and/or surgically unresectable disease has demonstrated poor local-regional control rates of 25%.[4]

Grade 3 and 4 toxicities, according to the Radiation Therapyn Oncology group and European Organization for research on the treatment of cancer (RTOG-EORTC), have been reported in patients undergoing neutron beam therapy, with significant complications such as osteoradionecrosis, optic neuritis/retinitis (blindness) and oral/pharyngeal-cutaneous fistulas occurring as high as 10% of the cases.[3,4]

The types of complications that may occur with radiotherapy are otitis externa, trismus, osteoradionecrosis, otitis media, transverse myelopathy, reduced hearing, skin breakdown, and meningitis. Some patients have more than one complication.[8]

Chemotherapy in management of salivary gland neoplasms

The role of chemotherapy in the management of salivary gland cancers is under study and in the budding stages. Various chemotherapeutic regimens are used currently for palliation of advanced tumors and there is no benefit for use in the induction or adjuvant setting.[3]

Suen and Johns had conducted a review of literature and surveyed experience of numerous institutions with chemotherapy for salivary gland malignancies. The overall response rate was found to be 42%.[6]

Kaplan et al, found that adenocarcinomas responded best to a combination of cisplatin, doxorubicin and 5-fluorouracil.[9]

Generally combination therapy is more effective against salivary gland tumors as compared to single-drug therapy. Airoldi et al, 2000, have concluded that the most effective drug regimens include cisplatin, paclitaxel, doxorubicin, 5-fluorouracil and epirubicin in different combinations.[6]

According to Jones AS et al, although salivary gland cancers show some response to various chemotherapeutic agents, these responses are rarely complete, are usually short-lived, and have not resulted in significant improvement in long-term survival.[10] A recent study indicated that the frequent expression of multidrug resistant genes by carcinoma of the salivary glands might be responsible for the low response rates to conventional chemotherapy.[11]

References

1. Buchholz TA, Laramore GE, Griffin BR, Koh WJ, Griffin TW. The role of fast neutron radiation therapy in the management of advanced salivary gland malignant neoplasms. Cancer. 1992;69:2779-88.
2. Hanna EY, Suen JY. The Parotid Neoplasm. Pensak ML (Ed). Controversies in Otolaryngology. Publication Thieme. Newyork. 2001;22(66):348-54.
3. Bell RB, Dierks EJ, Homer L, Potter BE. Management and outcome of patients with malignant salivary gland tumors. J Oral Maxillofac Surg. 2005;63:917-28.
4. Douglas JG, Koh WJ, Austin-Seymour M, Laramore GE. Treatment of salivary gland neoplasms with fast neutron radiotherapy. Arch Otolaryngol Head Neck Surg. 2003;129:944-8.

5. Langdon JD. Operative Maxillofacial surgery. Sublingual and Submandibular gland excision. Langdon JD, Patel MF (Eds). Chapman and Hall Medical, London. 1998;32:375-80.
6. Hanna EY, Suen JY. Malignant tumors of the salivary glands. Myers EN, Suen JY, Myers JN, Hanna EY, (Eds). Cancer of the head and neck. 4th edn. Saunders. 21.pp.475-510.
7. Henry LW, Blasko JC, Griffin TW, et al. Evolution of fast neutron teletherapy for advanced carcinomas of the major salivary glands. Cancer. 1979;44:814-8.
8. Jackson GL, Luna MA, Byers RM. Results of surgery alone and surgery combined with postoperative radiotherapy in the treatment of cancer of the parotid gland. 1983;146:497-500.
9. Kaplan MJ, Johns ME, Cantrell RW. Chemotherapy for salivary gland cancer. Otolaryngol Head Neck Surg. 1986;95:165-70.
10. Jones AS, Philips DE, Cook JA, et al. A randomized phase II trial of epirubicin and %-fluorouracil versus cisplatin in the palliation of advanced and recurrent malignant tumor of the salivary glands. Br J Cancer. 1993;67:112-4.
11. Uematsu T, Hasegawa T, Hiraoka BY, et al. Multidrug resistance gene 1 expression in salivary gland adenocarcinomas and oral squamous cell carcinomas. Int J Cancer. 2001;92:187-94.

Index

Page numbers followed by 'f' refer to figure and 't' refer to table

A

Ablative tumor surgery 85f
Acinic cell
   adenocarcinoma 147, 163
   carcinoma 32, 52
Acinous cell carcinoma 98, 100
Acute bacterial sialadenitis 54
Adenocarcinoma 32, 100
Adenoid cystic carcinoma 32, 52, 99,
      142, 145f, 146f, 163, 202f
Adenolymphoma 120
Adson and Ott incision 178f
Advantages of functional superficial
      parotidectomy 187
Alcoholic cirrhosis 31
American Joint Commission on
      Cancer 103
Angle of mandible 18
Anorexia 55
Antistaphylococcal penicillins 59
Aplasia 31
Appiani's incision 179f
Arteriography 49
Atresia 31
Auriculotemporal syndrome 214

B

Bacitracin 210
Ball in hand appearance 46f
Bartholin's
   duct 26
   gland 6
Basal cell
   adenocarcinoma 32
   adenoma 2, 32, 120
Bell's palsy 37
Benign
   epithelial tumors 32
   lymphoepithelial lesion of
      Godwin 74
   tumor of parotid 36f
Bicellular stem cell theory 91
Bimanual palpation of submandibular
      gland 38f
Blair's incision 179, 181f, 184f, 189f
Blood supply 16, 24, 26
Blossom tree appearance 45f
Branchless fruit laden tree appearance
      45f
Bulimia 55

C

Canalicular adenoma 2, 32, 123,
      124, 124f
Cannulation of
   duct 43f
   duct with PVC tube 86f
Carcinoma 63
   ex mixed tumor 152, 153
   ex pleomorphic adenoma 32, 154f
Carcinosarcoma 32, 152, 156
Carpal tunnel syndrome 78
Cavernous hemangioma 82
Cerebrospinal fluid 72
Chemotherapy in management of
      salivary gland neoplasms 218
Chronic bacterial sialadenitis 62
Classification of
   neoplasms 97
   tumors of salivary gland 32
Clear cell carcinoma 32, 160, 161f
Computed tomography 50
Cut section of
   mucoepidermoid carcinoma 134f
   pleomorphic adenoma 109
   Warthin's tumor 114f
Cystadenocarcinoma 32

Cystadenoma 32
Cystic fibrosis 55
Cysts 1, 31

D

Depression 55
Diabetes mellitus 31, 55
Dicloxacillin 59
Dilation of duct with lacrimal probe 43f
Distance of facial nerve pointers from surrounding landmarks 18
Distant metastasis 104
Doppler ultrasound 40, 42
Drawbacks of monitoring 21
Ductal
 anomalies 54
 papilloma 2, 32, 125
Ducts of gland 26
Dumbbell tumor 189f
 of parotid gland 9f, 107f

E

Endogenous hormones 91
Enlargement of gland 1, 31
Epidemic parotitis 70
Epithelial
 carcinoma 32, 162
 cells 98
 myoepithelial carcinoma 163f
Epstein-Barr viruses 90
Exanthematous fevers 54
Excision of
 neoplasms of cheek and lips 205
 palatal
  adenoid cystic carcinoma 204
  mucoepidermoid carcinoma 204
  pleomorphic adenomas 203
 sublingual gland 198
 tumor 203
Extent of
 gland 6, 21
 growth 34
 parotid gland 7f
External auditory canal 18

Extracapsular excision of submandibular salivary gland 199
Extracorporeal lithotripsy 69
Extravasation cysts 31

F

Facial
 artery 22
 nerve 182
  dissection 10f, 189f
  monitoring 20
  paralysis 37
  paresis or paralysis 213
  pointers 18f
  preservation 188
Fine needle aspiration cytopathology 40, 50
Fluorodeoxyglucose 49
Functional superficial parotidectomy 181, 186

G

Gallium scintigraphy 50
Gastrointestinal and hepatobiliary manifestations 78
General classification of salivary gland diseases 31
Gland
 morphology 8
 neoplasms 203
Glenoid process 12
Glossopharyngeal nerve 16
Glycopyrolate 213
Grading of mucoepidermoid carcinoma 136
Gutierrez incision 176f

H

Heerfordt's syndrome 37
Hemangioma 33
Hematogenous infections 54
Hematolymphoid tumors 33
Hematoma 212
Hemolytic anemia 73

Haemophilus influenzae 56
Hepatic failure 55
Hepatocyte growth factor 93
High grade mucoepidermoid
 carcinoma 139
Histogenesis of salivary gland
 neoplasms 97
HIV
 associated
  parotitis 55
  salivary gland disease 73
 parotitis 73
Hodgkin lymphoma 33
Hyperlipoproteinemia 55
Hyperuricemia 55
Hypothyroidism 55

I

Identification of
 facial nerve 16, 180, 184f
 tumor mass 181f
Incidence of salivary gland
 neoplasms 95
 tumors 96
Incision 206, 207
Incisional biopsy 40, 51
Inflammation of Wharton's
 duct 58f, 66f
Intermediate grade mucoepidermoid
 carcinoma 138, 138f
Intraductal papilloma 32, 130
Intraoral
 deep lobe tumor excision 187
 lesion 210f
Inverted ductal papilloma 32, 128,
 129f
Ionic aqueous solution 42
Irradiation of gland 85

J

Jeryl Lynn vaccine 72

K

Keratoconjunctivitis sicca 77

L

Large cell carcinoma 32
Liver failure 54
Local excision of parotid gland 180, 181
Loss of wrinkling of forehead 213f
Low-grade
 cribriform adenocarcinoma 32
 mucoepidermoid carcinoma 82,
  137, 137f
Lymphadenoma 32
Lymphoepithelial carcinoma 32, 164

M

Magnetic resonance imaging 50
Malignant
 epithelial tumors 32
 lymphoepithelial lesion 164
 mixed tumor 52, 152
 parotid tumor 37f
 salivary gland tumors 2
 tumor 37f
  of palatal salivary gland 39f
  of salivary glands 131
Management of
 acinic cell adenocarcinoma 152
 adenoid cystic carcinoma 146
 basal cell adenomas 122
 canalicular adenomas 125
 carcinoma ex-mixed tumor 155
 carcinosarcoma 157
 metastasizing mixed tumor 158
 mucocele over lip 82f
 mucoepidermoid carcinoma 139
 oncocytoma 120
 pleomorphic adenoma of
  palate 112
  parotid gland 111
  submandibular gland 112
 Warthin's tumor 116
Mandibular ramus and masseter
 muscle 6
Maxillary sinus 48f, 205f
McFee incision 194f
Metastasizing
 mixed tumor 152, 157
 pleomorphic adenoma 32

Methicillin 59
   resistant *Staphylococcus aureus* 56
Mikulicz's disease 31, 45, 74
Minor salivary gland 1, 38
   tumor 48*f*
Mixed tumor 98
Modified Blair's incision in adult 180*f*
Monomorphic adenoma 120
Mucicarmine stains 129
Mucinous adenocarcinoma 32
Mucoceles 80
   of lower lip and tongue 81*f*
Mucoepidermoid carcinoma 32, 52, 99, 131, 163
   of submandibular gland and minor gland of palate 133*f*
Mucous
   extravasation phenomenon 84*f*
   retention phenomenon 84*f*
   salivary glands 1
Multicellular theory 91
Multilobulated
   parotid tumor 36*f*
   tumor of tail of parotid 36*f*
Mumps 31, 70
Murine double minute 92
Mycobacterium
   avium-intracellulare 56
   tuberculosis 56
Mylohyoid muscle 64
Myocarditis 73
Myoepithelial
   carcinoma 32, 162
   cells 98
Myoepithelioma 2, 32

N

Necrotizing sialometaplasia 1, 31
Non-Hodgkin's lymphoma 63
Non-infectious inflammatory diseases 74
Non-neoplastic
   diseases 54
   disorders 54
Nutritional deficiency 31

O

Obstructive disorders of salivary glands 63
Oil-based solution 42
Oncocytic
   carcinoma 32
   tumors 100
Oncocytoma **32**, 117, 119*f*, 120
Opening of Stensen's duct 58
Orthopantomogram 40
Oxacillin 59
Oxyphilic adenoma 2, 120

P

Papillary cystadenoma lymphomatosum 113
Para-influenza virus 31
Parotid
   abscess 60*f*
   duct 12, 187
   gland 6
      stones 65
      swelling 57*f*
   lesions 80
   neoplasm 36*f*
   papilla 66*f*
   stone removal 69
   tumor 35, 48*f*
Parotidectomy 182, 191, 193
Parotidomandibulectomy 191
Partial
   maxillectomy 206
   obstruction of gland 64
   superficial parotidectomy 187
Pathophysiology of salivary gland tumors 92
Pectoralis major myocutaneous 195
Periodic acid-Schiff stain 129, 135, 145, 163
Pes anserinus 15
Plasmacytosis 73
Pleomorphic adenoma 2, 32, 50, 105, 110*f*, 163
   of minor salivary gland of palate 108*f*

of palatal minor salivary
glands 39f
of palate 203f
of parotid gland 106f
of submandibular gland 107f
Polyarteritis nodosa 76
Polyarthritis 73
Polymorphous low grade
adenocarcinoma 32, 150f
Polymyositis 76
Positron emission tomography 40,
49, 50
Preservation of facial nerve 181
Primary
biliary cirrhosis 77
squamous cell carcinoma 158
Proliferating cell nuclear antigen 93
Pseudolymphoma 63
Pseudomonas aeruginosa 56
Pterygoid plates 48

R
Radical
excision of neoplasms of
submandibular 202
neck dissection 194f
Radionucleotide scanning 40, 46
Radiotherapy 140
for head and neck cancer 55
Ranula 26, 31, 82
in floor of mouth 83f
Recurrent pleomorphic adenoma in
child 112f
Redon and Vaillant and Laudenbach
incision 177f
Regional lymph nodes 104
Relation of facial nerve with parotid
gland 11f
Renal failure 55
Respiratory tract involvement 78
Retention cysts 31
Retromandibular incision 60f
Rheumatoid arthritis 76

S
Salivary
caruncle 58f
duct carcinoma 32
fistula 84, 213
gland 1, 6, 62
dysfunction 1, 31
tumors 1
Samengo incision 178f
Scleroderma 76, 77
Sclerotherapy 74
Sebaceous
adenoma 32
carcinoma 32, 163
lymphadenocarcinoma 32
Serous salivary glands 1
Severe dehydration 55
Sialadenoma papilleferum 32, 125,
127f
Sialoblastoma 32
Sialographic appearances 46f
Sialography 40, 42, 43
Sialolith of Wharton's duct 66f
Sialolithiasis 64
Sialorrhea 31
Sjögren's
disease 74
syndrome 31, 55, 74-79
Skin incision and exposure of
gland 176
Small
cell carcinoma 32, 167
lymphangioma 82
Soft tissue tumors 33
Squamous cell carcinoma 32, 99
Staphylococcus aureus 56, 62
Stensen's duct 12, 58, 59, 64, 187
Streptococcus
pneumoniae 56
pyogenes 56
viridans 62
Structures traversing gland 14
Styloid process 18

Sublingual
  caruncle in floor of mouth 66f
  glands 25
  salivary gland 38, 202, 202f
Submandibular
  duct 24
  gland 21, 23f, 67f, 189f, 198, 200f
    tumor 37, 39f
  incision 199f, 200f, 201f
Subtotal maxillectomy 205f
Superficial
  lobe 36f
  parotidectomy 63, 181, 184f
  relations of submandibular
    gland 25f
Surgical management of
  minor salivary 203
  parotid neoplasms 175
  submandibular and sublingual
    neoplasms 198
Surgical pathology of salivary gland
  neoplasms 102
Systemic lupus erythematosus 76, 77

T

Technetium scintigraphy 50
Total
  maxillectomy 188, 207
  parotidectomy 81, 194f
Transoral surgical management of
  submandibular calculus 68f
Transverse section of parotid gland 8f
Trismus 212
True malignant mixed tumor 152
Tumor
  of palatal minor salivary
    gland 205f
  of salivary glands 1, 31
  resection 180
  rupture 188
Tympanomastoid suture 18
Typical parotid tumor 36f

U

Uncontrolled hemorrhage 188
Undifferentiated
  carcinomas 164
  large cell carcinomas 164, 166
Unilateral acute bacterial parotitis 57f
Upper trapezius myocutaneous
  flap 195
Uremia 54
Urinary tract involvement 78
Uveoparotitis 75

V

Viral infections of salivary glands 70
von Ebner's glands 6

W

Warthin's tumor 2, 32, 113, 115f, 116,
  117, 120, 125, 181
Weber-Ferguson incision 210f
Wharton's duct 41f, 67f, 200

X

Xeropthalmia 77
Xerostomia 31, 79

Z

Zidovudine 74
Zygomatic arch 191